Hypnosis in the Management of Sleep Disorders

Hypnosis in the Management of Sleep Disorders combines history and medical science to show that the use of hypnosis and hypnotic techniques is effective in the treatment of sleep disorders – and that this is increasingly validated through modern tools (computers, fMRI images). Dr. Kohler and Kurz show readers that hypnosis and hypnotic techniques are not to be feared or avoided, but that their use can contribute to effective, non-intrusive, and cost-effective approaches to the treatment of sleep problems. This volume is a much-needed reference for therapists and their patients alike on how hypnosis can be helpful in the treatment of certain sleep disorders.

William C. Kohler, M.D., was among the leading medical doctors practicing sleep medicine in the United States. A graduate of the University of Florida's Medical School in Gainesville, Florida, he was board-certified in sleep medicine, pediatrics, and neurology (with special competence in child neurology). Dr. Kohler was also a trained, experienced user of hypnosis in medical treatment. As an approved consultant in clinical hypnosis with the American Society of Clinical Hypnosis, he was one of the earliest and most respected experts in this field. Dr. Kohler died only weeks after the complete manuscript was delivered to the publisher.

Peter J. Kurz, a professional writer, translator, and photographer living in Pennsylvania, co-authored *Hypnosis in the Management of Sleep Disorders*.

Hypnosis in the Management of Sleep Disorders

William C. Kohler, M.D., and
Peter J. Kurz

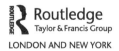
Routledge
Taylor & Francis Group

LONDON AND NEW YORK

First published 2017
by Routledge
711 Third Avenue, New York, NY 10017

and by Routledge
2 Park Square, Milton Park, Abingdon, Oxon, OX14 4RN

Routledge is an imprint of the Taylor & Francis Group, an informa business

© 2018 Taylor & Francis

Library of Congress Cataloging in Publication Data
Names: Kurz, Peter J., author. | Kohler, William C., author.
Title: Hypnosis in the management of sleep disorders / by Peter J. Kurz and William C. Kohler.
Description: New York, NY : Routledge, 2017. Includes bibliographical references and index.
Identifiers: LCCN 2017004191| ISBN 9781138062283 (hbk : alk. paper) | ISBN 9781138062290 (pbk : alk. paper) | ISBN 9781315161709 (ebk)
Subjects: LCSH: Sleep disorders—Alternative treatment. | Hypnotism—Therapeutic use.
Classification: LCC RC547 .K87 2017 DDC 616.8/498—dc23
LC record available at https://lccn.loc.gov/2017004191

ISBN: 978-1-138-06228-3 (hbk)
ISBN: 978-1-138-06229-0 (pbk)
ISBN: 978-1-315-16170-9 (ebk)

Typeset in Sabon
by Swales & Willis, Exeter, Devon, UK

WCK: *To my wonderful wife of 52 years, Barbara B. Kohler, without whose tireless assistance and support this book would never have been completed* (written upon completion of the manuscript and its submission to the publisher on September 29, 2014).

PJK: *With love and thanks to my wife Corriene V. Kurz, M.D., for her constant inspiration and patience.*

Contents

Preface

More than half a century ago the two authors of this book were high school classmates in New Jersey. Somehow, during or after Dr. Law's Latin class, we became deeply involved in a conversation about how wasteful it was to sleep. That same day we continued our conversation in the Kohler family's kitchen . . . and the next days and weeks as well. We even devised steps by which we could experiment with potential ways to "compress" sleep and to "reduce the amount of time" we had to spend sleeping. Why is it, we asked, that we must spend one-third of our lives asleep? And we couldn't find a good answer . . .

We agreed on and reluctantly admitted the need for somewhere between six and ten hours every night because our "research" had demonstrated to both of us that we wouldn't "feel good" below or above that range – certainly not on less than six hours. So the question before us was: How could we simultaneously reduce the number of hours slept while maintaining the feeling of mental alertness and physical well-being which – we agreed – we enjoyed when afforded the luxury of around eight hours of sleep? One experiment still remembered vividly from way back in the last millennium is our (unsuccessful) attempt at trying to go through the equivalent of a "full night's" sleep over a "reduced" period of an arbitrarily picked three hours – in a warm bath. Maybe sleeping for three hours in a full bath tub instead of our beds would provide us with a good night's sleep without the "cost" of eight hours.

Another "experiment" consisted of a gradual reduction by something like 15 minutes every night over a period of weeks of the amount of sleep we allowed ourselves (neither of us can remember the exact details). The idea was to see if we could adjust without significant adverse effects and reach the desired target number (we can't remember what that was, but perhaps it was somewhere around four hours a night). Well . . . that didn't work out either. The way we remember, after a few weeks we stopped the experiment because we were too tired to function.

Both of us moved on to college and Bill continued at the University of Florida's medical school in Gainesville. His interest in the fascinating issues of sleep, dreaming, and sleep medicine not only continued but increased.

Bill's interest in sleep medicine flourished and he dedicated his life to the pursuit of this nascent, rapidly growing specialty. While in medical school he published a paper in the February, 1968 issue of *The Journal of Pediatrics* (Appendix A). "Sleep Patterns in 2-Year-Old Children" is important for several reasons. For the first time it described the sleep patterns of two-year-olds and the related physiological changes in their brains. In addition to its several findings, it established a baseline against which future changes in sleep patterns could be measured. The association of rapid eye movement (REM) sleep and dreaming in two-year-olds was also described for the first time.

This book is an outgrowth of and is based on Dr. Kohler's conclusions about the physiology and clinical importance of sleep, derived from his decades of clinical experience in the practice of sleep medicine. Added to that are his more than two decades of experience in the use of hypnosis and hypnotic techniques in the effective treatment of certain sleep disorders.

We feel that hypnosis can be an important, effective, non-invasive treatment for certain sleep disorders. It is self-empowering and without major side-effects. Aside from the obvious benefits to the patient, greater usage will lead to a better understanding of hypnosis as a medical procedure, which will in turn lead to more scientific attention and focus on additional research.

William C. Kohler, M.D.
Peter J. Kurz
Tampa, Florida, 2014

Acknowledgments

The assistance of Sharon B. Henrich, librarian at Florida Hospital Tampa, in obtaining dozens of journal and book articles, is greatly appreciated.

Jeanne C. Brewster, Customer Service Representative with Copyright Clearance Services, was instrumental in obtaining the necessary permissions to reproduce figures.

We are grateful for the assistance received from the staff of Princeton University's Firestone Library, its Seeley G. Mudd Manuscript Library, the Library of Congress in Washington, D.C., and the Washington County Free Library (WCFL). In particular, at WCFL we acknowledge with thanks the professional and always cheerful help of Tammy Gantz and Louise Snurr.

The authors thank the valuable contribution and constant support of Elizabeth Kohler, RPSGT, RST, who was enormously helpful during the various phases of this project. Ms. Kohler worked with Dr. Kohler, her father, as Technical Director of the Florida Sleep Institute. She helped compile information for this book, especially in locating and identifying sleep records and with the tracking down of information for figures which demonstrated various points in the work.

In addition the authors thank Lance Wobus of Taylor & Francis, for understanding our vision and sharing his insights related to our work's importance, relevance and quality. Similarly, after Dr. Kohler's death, I am grateful for the encouragement and support received for this work from Kay Conerly, also of Taylor & Francis. At Routledge, I'm immensely grateful to George Zimmar and Meira Bienstock for their guidance, help and for making this work possible. Also for the assistance received from Lillian Rand, Editor, Taylor & Francis in New York. During the final three months of production, the very professional and able technical and editorial help received from Kristin Susser, Julie Willis (Swales & Willis) and Liz Williams was invaluable and motivating. Their perspicacious, patient, yet always prompt responses, are greatly appreciated.

Author Biographies

William C. Kohler, M.D., was the founder and medical director of the Florida Sleep Institute. He earned his A.B. at Oberlin College and his M.D. at the University of Florida College of Medicine. He was board-certified in Sleep Medicine, Neurology with special competence in Child Neurology, Pediatrics, as well as Electroencephalography and Neurophysiology. He studied hypnotherapy under the guidance of Dr. Bernauer "Fig" Newton and was an Approved Consultant in Clinical Hypnosis with the American Society of Clinical Hypnosis. He was a spokesperson for the American Academy of Sleep Medicine (AASM) and chairman of the AASM accreditation committee. His 1968 article "Sleep Patterns in 2-Year-Old Children," published in *The Journal of Pediatrics* was the first description of the association of REM sleep with dreaming and the description of sleep parameters for that age group. He was often a guest speaker at numerous conferences both in the United States and abroad.

Born in Budapest, **Peter J. Kurz** earned a B.A. in Politics from Princeton University (with a Certificate in European Civilization) and an M.A. in Portuguese and Spanish literature from the University of Florida, Gainesville. After teaching Brazilian Portuguese to Peace Corps volunteers, he attended Officer Candidate School in Newport, Rhode Island, and was commissioned an Ensign, US Navy. During his professional career as a journalist, international banker, and a strategic and financial consultant with major US consulting firms, he worked in and visited more than 80 countries, dabbled in nine languages and, today, remains comfortable in four. As a member of Citicorp/Citibank's international staff he has lived and worked in New York City, London, Beirut, Athens, Jeddah, Houston, and Madrid. He continues to write and to translate.

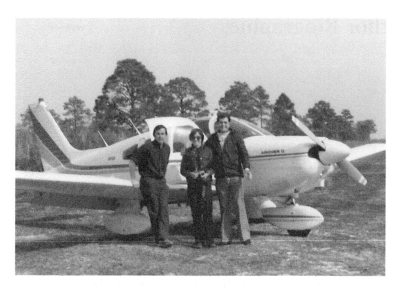

Figure 0.1 Family photograph taken during the 1970s. From left to right: Peter J. Kurz, Barbara B. Kohler, and her husband, Dr. William C. Kohler. By then, both Dr. and Mrs. Kohler had earned their pilot's licenses and this photograph was taken at the Kohler family airstrip in Keaton Beach, Florida (still active today as private airfield 6FL4). (See Plate 1.)

In Memoriam Dr. William C. Kohler

Dr. W. McDowell Anderson

PULMONARY CRITICAL CARE AND SLEEP MEDICINE,
JAMES A. HALEY VA HOSPITAL, TAMPA, FLORIDA

Dr. William C. Kohler, M.D., 72, of Brooksville, Florida passed away on October 15, 2014. He and his wife Barbara entered Oberlin College in Ohio together and were married before their graduation in 1964. Dr. Kohler earned his M.D. in 1968 at the University of Florida, College of Medicine, where he also continued his studies in Medical, Pediatric, and Neurology (Adult & Pediatric) training (1968–1973). He served as a Major in the U.S. Air Force after which he returned to a faculty position at the University of Florida.

A love for the wild and rural life led him to establish a private practice, The Sleep Center of Montana, in Billings, Montana. Moving his family back to Florida, he established the Florida Sleep Institute in Brooksville. However, he could not shake his academic roots and was also recruited to establish the Pediatric Sleep Center at University Community Hospital (now Florida Hospital, Tampa). Additionally, from 2009 to 2014 he established and maintained the pediatric sleep training component for the Sleep Fellowship Program at the Morsani College of Medicine, University of South Florida. From 1986, Dr. Kohler was an active member of the American Academy of Sleep Medicine (AASM).

These accomplishments all pale in relation to Bill/Dad/Grandad's (as many of us know him) accomplishments as a husband, father, grandfather, friend, and a distinguished community and local church leader. This is how he would have wanted most to be remembered. Always the quiet and consummate gentleman, he would volunteer his time and expertise to anyone in need.

(The above excerpts are from a tribute first published in the *Journal of Clinical Sleep Medicine* (2015) January 15, 11 (1): 83.)

1 Introduction

This book was written for anyone interested in learning more about sleep and how an unappreciated, underused, and misunderstood technique – hypnosis – can be a medically sound and effective way to treat a number of sleep disorders.

The authors feel that hypnosis can be a non-invasive, important addition to the ways in which certain sleep disorders can be treated effectively and with fewer side-effects than other alternatives. Aside from the obvious benefits to the patient, greater usage will lead to a better understanding of hypnosis as a medical procedure, which will in turn lead to more scientific attention and focus on additional research.

Our most important goal is to provide an accurate and readable overview of the fields of sleep and the use of hypnosis in sleep medicine. The authors hope that this book will provide basic information useful to practitioners in the medical field as well as the interested general public. It is neither a "self-help" book nor a medical textbook. Rather than being an encyclopedic compilation of data and case studies the authors tried to offer a book that provides an easy-to-read but useful mix of historical and scientific background. To make the book readable, when needed our notes are at the end of each chapter, not disruptive to the flow of the text, yet easy to find in the context of each chapter and its major topic.

A second objective is to provide a useful, credible listing of references and resources for the reader who is or becomes more interested in one or all of these important – and very much related – topics. The reader who wants to learn more about aspects covered in the text can find them in the notes or through the resources sections at the end of the book (Appendix D).

This work should be particularly useful to those who are interested in or need a book on the new science of sleep and in new forms of treatment for certain sleep disorders. Dr. Kohler believes that hypnosis and hypnotic techniques should be at the forefront when considering treatment for sleep disorders. It may be a clarion call to professionals in the medical field, in the field of hypnosis, existing patients or others, perhaps, who have family members, friends or co-workers who could benefit from the treatment of sleep disorders through hypnotic techniques.

At the turn of the nineteenth century, between 1890 and around 1920, several major developments and discoveries radically changed our understanding of the brain and the function of sleep. Dr. J. Allan Hobson, a professor and psychiatrist at Harvard Medical School, narrows the critical period even further:

> If we were asked to identify the time frame in which the psychological and neuro-physiological study of the brain/mind took on its current "modern" form it would be the decade between 1890 and 1900. In that decade three important developments set the science of sleep and dreaming on its current course.
>
> (Hobson and Wohl 2005)

In the following chapters this book will elaborate on these and other "important developments." We will provide an outline of how, in a parallel course and affected by these developments, our understanding of hypnosis also changed significantly. This has led to the increased and effective use of hypnosis in the medical treatment of certain sleep disorders that will also be part of this book's message.

In summary, the four messages the authors hope to convey to readers of this book can be stated as follows.

First, there is a new "science of brain" which continues to change and evolve as a result of unprecedented technical and related medical advances. This enhanced understanding of how the brain functions is interrelated with our understanding of other areas such as sleep, dreaming, and hypnosis.

Second, we now know more about sleep and its function and effect on human well-being than has ever been known before. Since the development of electroencephalographic technology (EEG) and the introduction of polysomnograms (PSGs) plus the discovery of rapid eye movement (REM) state sleep (in 1953), we have reached a new definition of sleep and of its many functions. We now know that sleep is not merely the "absence of wakefulness," that the brain continues to be active at a very high rate even during sleep, and that sleep provides humans with numerous benefits far beyond just rest.

Third, these same instruments and a more sophisticated and accurate understanding of our brain and the nature of sleep have also clarified to a certain extent our understanding of the nature and function of dreaming.

Finally, also on a parallel track of rapidly occurring new discoveries is our understanding of hypnosis and the effectiveness with which hypnotic techniques can be used in the medical treatment of patients. This track is affected and influenced by the parallel developments in the fields of mind, sleep, and dream science.

Our hope is that this work will reach a wide audience and, therefore, will stimulate additional interest, foment more research, and for many more patients will lead to better treatment.

Recent advances in our understanding of how the brain functions have been so rapid and numerous that it is difficult to keep pace in our understanding of what has been discovered and what these discoveries mean. The historical background we will cover, our concomitant current understanding, and the practical results from which we benefit today are only a beginning.

The pace of new developments is accelerating and the findings and consequences are – literally – mind boggling! With the technological advances of the last decades – particularly in computer science, optics, and radiology – valuable and unique research constantly results in major, at times surprising, new findings. This research is no longer limited to a few distinguished and well-known academic and scientific centers. The major research and academic centers of Western Europe, Japan, and North America will continue to amaze us with their new and astonishing discoveries and surprising announcements. But valuable – routine as well as extraordinary – research is going on throughout the world. And, equally importantly, it is shared and dissipated to all corners of the globe, more rapidly and in greater numbers than ever in human history. The authors believe that this will continue at what may become an even faster pace.

The authors also believe that this will introduce a new era – *an exciting new future* – in the treatment of sleep disorders. As we unlock the scientific mysteries of the brain, of sleep, dreaming, and hypnosis, the authors believe that the results that Dr. Kohler has already seen will be enhanced, leveraged, and multiplied through the better use of already existing as well as through the future use of yet unimaginable tools and techniques.

But first, before we dive into the new science of sleep and a more detailed discussion of why and how hypnosis is expected to become an effective way to treat numerous diseases – including sleep disorders – we will explore in more detail the very basic topics of *what is sleep?* And *what is hypnosis?*

Reference

Hobson, J. Allan and Hellmut Wohl. 2005. *From Angels to Neurones: Art and The New Science of Dreaming*. Special Edition. Fidenza: Mattioli 1885.

2 What is Sleep?

> I don't understand what you say, replied Sancho; I only know for sure that as long as I'm asleep I have neither fear nor hope, neither work, nor glory; and praise be to whoever invented sleep, the very cloak that covers all human thoughts, food that removes hunger, water that drives away thirst, the fire that warms the cold, cold that tempers heat, and the universal currency with which all can be acquired, the weight and balance which makes a shepherd the equal of a king and the fool the same as a wise man. According to what I've heard, there is only one thing wrong with sleep and it is that it's like death; there is very little difference between the sleeping person and the dead.
>
> (Cervantes, 2010, *Don Quixote*, Part II, Chapter LXVIII)[1]

All of us "know" what sleep is. This state called sleep may be mysterious and its purpose may be puzzling, but all humans experience it for periods of more or less the same length of time and within quite predictable, cyclical intervals. Yet we struggle when asked to describe and to define it. Why? After all, since recorded history there is evidence that healthy humans spend around one-third of their lives in this state – sleeping. Whether in Africa, Asia, Europe, everywhere on earth and now also in space, today as thousands of years ago, females and males, young and old, tall, short, overweight or thin – for all sleep is a most essential and universal need and practice.

Imagine how this would look to very different outside visitors observing us for the first time, perhaps imaginary aliens from another planet: regularly, everywhere, animals stop at predictable intervals, assume an apparently inactive, passive state, and do not emerge for an equally predictable, specific period. This is precisely how our ancestors began to study sleep and in their notes or drawings left us a record of their varied conclusions, often based on very careful observation but always tinted by their environment, their philosophies of life and death, and, of course, a fertile imagination.

What is Sleep? Attempts to Depict, Describe, and Define

But what really *is* sleep? The truth is that we still don't know. Because it is so universal, essential to life, and predictable, also because for millennia it has been almost exclusively a nighttime event, many easy conclusions and superficial definitions emerged. We could only see the outward results of something we labeled sleep. We were not able to "touch" or otherwise document any hard physical evidence of how such a state came about. Interestingly, several cultures have used and continue to use the exact same word for "sleep" and "dreaming." One example is Spanish, illustrated by the great Cervantes in his story of the adventures of Don Quixote and his squire, Sancho Panza. The Spanish equivalent of the English "sleep" is *sueño*, as is "dream." Consequently it is impossible for a translation into English of the passage quoted at the beginning of this chapter to reflect completely the nuances which Cervantes observed and knowingly inserted. The comparison Sancho makes when describing the "only fault" or negative aspect of *sueño* – that "it's like death" – could be a reference to either or both "sleep" and "dream" (*Oxford Spanish Dictionary* 2003, 780).[2]

At the beginning of the twenty-first century we know more than we have ever known about the brain and the states of sleep, dreaming, and hypnosis, but even so we have only begun to scratch the surface. The four are related and intertwined and the more we learn about each the more we are awed by how one touches the other. It is precisely the rapid exchange of new discoveries and information in each of these sciences that propels and accelerates the phenomenal progress we now see in our understanding of each.

Most definitions of sleep are incomplete, inadequate, or outright inaccurate. Because our understanding of the scientific basis was missing until very recently, such definitions have always been circumstantial, without the benefit of the neurological and physiological information which we began to amass during the past century or so. In defining sleep, the *Oxford English Dictionary* (OED) reflects the difficulty in attempting to be complete, precise, and accurate. In defining "sleep," even the Compact Edition fills a beginning page, moves through two additional pages, and finishes at the end of the fourth page. The next word – "sleeper" – begins two full pages of additional English words beginning with some form of "sleep" (sleepiness, sleepwalker, finally stopping at "sleepy"). The most significant first definition of sleep (the noun) is:

1. a. The unconscious state or condition regularly and naturally assumed by man and animals, during which the activity of the nervous system is almost or entirely suspended, and recuperation of its powers takes place; slumber, repose. Also, a similar state artificially induced, as hypnotic (or magnetic) sleep.

    (*Oxford English Dictionary* 2014, "sleep")

Adding: "The word is further applied to the more inert condition of certain animals during hibernation." The verb "to sleep" is defined primarily (1.a.) as "To take repose by the natural suspension of consciousness; to be in the state of sleep; to slumber."

Dictionary definitions are not always accurate. The authors (WCK and PJK) believe that by the end of this work the reader will find this first definition to be inaccurate and oversimplified. It is interesting to read OED's fourth definition related to what appears to be a universal linkage of "sleep" with "death" and dying: "4. Fig[urative] a. "The repose of death" (Usually with qualifying terms or phrases). To put to sleep, to kill, esp. painlessly." Another version by OED offers the following: "4. A state compared to or resembling sleep, such as death or complete silence or stillness" (*Oxford English Dictionary* 2014, "sleep").

As will be mentioned in later pages, our departure from waking consciousness at regular intervals for hours of "sleep" leads to major changes in brain wave activity and many physiological functions. Significant differences occur during the two major sleep stages, which will also be defined later. Sleep is a period of reduced motoric activity and of decreased responsiveness to external stimuli. But we have learned through modern scientific studies and with the help of modern techniques that the activity of the brain continues at a very high level even during sleep. However, first, let us look at sleep as most of humanity saw it for thousands of years, through the eyes of artists, storytellers, and writers.

What is Sleep? Artists and Writers Search for an Answer

For thousands of years, roughly until the beginning of the twentieth century, our understanding of sleep was entirely through perspicacious observation and inspired, talented depiction through words and art. Such works of art, literature, and philosophy have been created since the beginning of recorded history. The phenomenon of sleep has always been of great interest and concern. This interest is reflected through the history of ancient civilizations, whether passed down as beliefs or stories that were later recorded, whether carved in caves, out of stone, or passed on to us through numerous other ways. Of that small portion which was recorded, most of the earliest were probably lost or destroyed by age, disasters, or wars. This is precisely what makes the volume and variety of what survived, what we can still read and see today, so remarkable.

A brief summary is inadequate since it can't possibly convey the variety of interpretations offered. Even more than most of us, writers and artists everywhere have always been fascinated by "sleep" and "dreams"; they have found them to be inspiring topics for an enormous body of equally fascinating literary and artistic work. In addition to their sheer numbers, perhaps even more astounding is the variety with which these *leitmotifs* have been approached. Of course, the desire to categorize, to sort, to find meaning, and to try to identify and predict purpose have always been present. What made many of these so different from each other was their context, their specific environment, and the influence of others equally engaged in observing, studying, and distilling "the essence" of "What is Sleep?"

In English, among the deepest and most celebrated words attempting to define at least a few aspects of sleep are the following from Shakespeare, in Hamlet's soliloquy:

> . . . To die: to sleep;
> No more; and, by a sleep to say we end
> The heartache and the thousand natural shocks
> That flesh is heir to, 'tis a consummation
> Devoutly to be wish'd. To die, to sleep;
> To sleep: perchance to dream: ay, there's the rub;
> For in that sleep of death what dreams may come
> When we have shuffled off this mortal coil,
> Must give us pause . . .
> (Shakespeare, *Hamlet*, Act III, Scene 1)

Another early written record of the genesis of sleep is found in the second chapter of the Book of Genesis:

> 21   And the LORD God caused a deep sleep to fall upon Adam, while he slept: and he took one of his ribs, and closed up the flesh instead thereof;
> (*The Holy Bible, King James Version* 1988, Genesis 2: 21)

Implicit in this passage is an understanding of different kinds of sleep, one of which is "a deep sleep," and clearly stated is that this *deep sleep* was caused by "the LORD God." In the Gospels of the New Testament, among the very few references to Jesus Christ asleep is the episode describing a violent storm during a crossing of the Sea of Galilee. Three of the four gospels include this episode and describe it in a similar way. In Chapter 4, Mark wrote:

> 37   And there arose a great storm of wind, and the waves beat into the ship, so that the ship was now full.
> 38   And he was in the hinder part of the ship, asleep on the cushion; and they awake him and say unto him, "Master, carest thou not that we perish?"
> 39   And he arose and rebuked the wind, and said unto the sea, "Peace! Be still!" And the wind ceased, and there was a great calm.
> (*The Holy Bible, King James Version* 1988,
> Mark 4: 37–39)

One of the many reasons why the gospel writers included this story may have been to record the unusual conditions during which Jesus slept. In times of danger, especially outdoors, most people have difficulty falling asleep and, if already asleep, most will wake up. Among the prerequisites for good and deep sleep was a quiet, dark, comfortable environment. Even if tired at the end of a long day, the disciples were probably awake and unable to sleep because they were afraid and stressed, concerned about their safety, perhaps cold and wet. The contrast with Jesus being able to sleep is telling.

The association of death with sleep – and the concomitant fear – can also be illustrated through the first four lines of the still popular classic children's bedtime prayer:

> Now I lay me down to sleep,
> I pray thee Lord my soul to keep,
> If I shall die before I wake,
> I pray the Lord my soul to take. Amen.
>
> (*The New England Primer*, 1784)

Among the sleep-related stories that left their mark on the art and litera-ture of many countries in Europe and the Middle East is the story of the Seven Sleepers of Ephesus. It tells the tale of seven young Christian men who decided to escape persecution during the time of Roman Emperor Decius (circa 250 AD) by taking refuge in a cave near Ephesus. According to most narratives, eventually they fell asleep and allegedly slept for approximately 309 years. For almost 1,500 years thereafter their story and legend have been perpetuated through the best-known religious and lay writings, numerous works of art, and a variety of coffins and relics from Ephesus to France (and even locations in Africa). The story is mentioned in the *Roman Martyrology*, the Byzantine calendar, and many others, which influenced still others. At one point half the world's population knew of the long sleep of the seven. The vocabulary of many European languages still includes sleep-related words connected to the Seven Sleepers. In German, Dutch, Swedish, Norwegian, and Danish there are words for oversleeping which, apparently, originated from this story. This derivation goes beyond the Indo-European languages: in Hungarian *hétalvó* (literally a "seven-sleeper," or one who sleeps for an entire week) is a colloquial reference to someone who oversleeps or is usually drowsy (Fortescue 1909).[3]

Cervantes includes several passages in *Don Quijote* (in English: *Don Quixote*: Cervantes, 2003) that reflect the difficulty of proper sleep when concerned with problems of one kind or another. Sancho, the uneducated squire with limited ambitions and focused on simple, earthly needs, usu-ally sleeps long and well. His "noble" master, stressed and constantly preoccupied by a never-ending list of obligations and obstacles – real and imagined – can't ever seem to get a good night's sleep. Chapter 70 in Part II is introduced with a comment about how Sancho was invited by his master to sleep in his more comfortable, luxurious quarters:

> Sancho slept that night in a cot in the same chamber with Don Quixote, a thing he would have gladly excused if he could, for he knew very well that with questions and answers his master would not let him sleep, and he was in no humor for talking much . . .

Sancho is right in his premonition and, eventually, is forced to address the issue directly:

> "so I beg of your worship to let me sleep and not ask me any more questions, unless you want me to throw myself out of the window."
> "Sleep, Sancho my friend," said Don Quixote, "if the pin prodding and pinches thou has received and the snacks administered to thee will let thee."
> (Ormsby 2011, Part II, Chapter 20)

In another passage, Don Quixote contrasts Sancho's wonderful talent for falling asleep with his own apparent inability to do so:

> "Well then, let us turn to sleep and let's sleep during the little time that's left of the night and God shall wake us up in the morning."
> —You go to sleep, Sancho – replied Don Quixote –, you who were born to sleep; but I who was born to stand vigil, will spend the time left from now to the morning with my thoughts, and I will turn them into the song which, without your having realized, I composed in my mind.
> — It looks to me – answered Sancho – that the thoughts that lead to write verse aren't much. Compose however your honor wishes and I'll sleep as much as I can.
> (Ormsby 2011, Part LXVIII)[4]

Through the "Sleep of the Poor," the celebrated Mexican muralist Diego Rivera shows a group of children, women, and men peacefully asleep despite what may be less than ideal circumstances. Part of a fresco painted in this portion shows the group huddled together in a loving composition. Without beds, mats, or hammocks – let alone individual bedrooms – the group appears to be sleeping, carefree.

We inherited one of the most loved and lasting stories of the origins of both sleep and dreams from the Greeks. Hypnos, the god of sleep, according to Greek mythology, made his home in a dark, silent cave where he lived with his mother Night (*Nyx* in Greek) and twin brother, Thanatos (peaceful death). Their three sisters, the Keres, were associated with violent death and usually much feared as female death spirits.

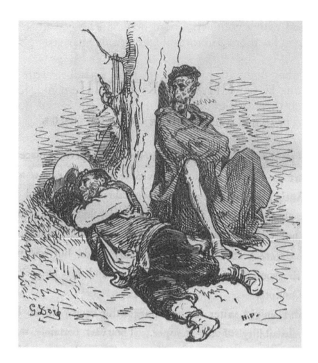

Figure 2.1 Illustration by the French painter and illustrator, Paul Gustave Doré (1832–1883). This image of a sleeping Sancho Panza next to an exhausted but awake Don Quixote is at the end of Part II, Chapter LXVII. Reproduced through Project Gutenberg Ebook of *The History of Don Quixote*, Volume II, Complete, by Miguel de Cervantes).

According to the Greeks, a river flows through or around the cave. Not the better known River Styx, the river of death that had to be crossed over to afterlife according to the Egyptians, but the River Lethe, from the plain of Lethe in Hades. Sometimes this river was mentioned as the river of unmindfulness, sometimes of forgetfulness, and some translations mention that its murmuring was said to induce drowsiness. Legends record that thought was given to the installation of some sort of gate at the entrance but this was vetoed, to avoid a potential creaking sound which could disturb sleep (Hypnos). Somehow even so the cave preserved both silence and darkness. According to the same stories, poppies grew at the entrance and clear, delicate images of these can still be seen today depicted on many Greek vases that have survived. It was a mysterious, feared place from which even Zeus, the mythological king of gods, stayed away.

Later, the Greek myths were adopted and translated by the Romans and the Greek Hypnos became the Latin Somnus, or Sopor, while Thanatos became known throughout the Roman Empire as Mors. From the eighth

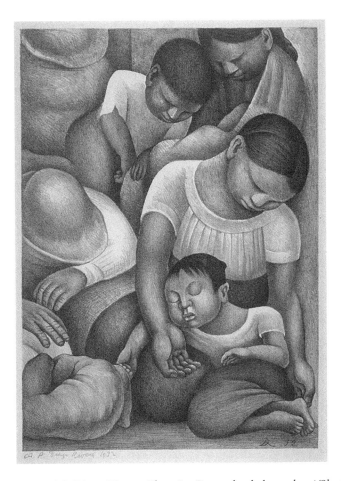

Figure 2.2 Diego Rivera, *El sueño (La noche de los pobres)/Sleep (The Night of the Poor)*. 1932. Lithograph, 22 5/8 × 15 7/8 inches. © 2014 Banco de México Diego Rivera Frida Kahlo Museums Trust, Mexico, D.F./Artists Rights Society (ARS), New York. (Reprinted with permission, Collection of the Madison Museum of Contemporary Art. Gift of Rudolph and Louise Langer.)

century BC through the first century AD, these stories continued in various versions perpetuated in the works by the great poets and writers of Greece, from Homer's *Iliad* to *The Orphic Hymns*. For the next 2,000 years they further inspired the most talented and best-known writers in Western civilization. And, of course, they also became the *leitmotif* and themes for the most admired artists who may have read the original stories in Greek and Latin, but most likely became familiar with the richness and variety of the themes through the many translations into all European as well as many other languages.

Today our own English vocabulary is replete with words derived from these Greek and Roman origins: hypnosis, hypnotic, hypnotize, somnolent, somnambulism, mortified. The Romance languages have an even larger and richer collection of words from these common roots.

The surviving works of art and literature that have touched upon so many facets of the nightly process we call sleep describe a great variety of needs, concerns, and solutions. For instance, when and where to sleep? For good sleep Hypnos required a cave that was dark and silent.

Centuries and a continent away, in real life today, hammocks are the preferred nightly resting place for a very large percentage of the Central and South American population. Today, for comfort, portability, and habit on board the regularly scheduled *gaiolas* (riverboats) that ply the Amazon River virtually all passengers – 300 or more travelers at a time – sleep on their own hammocks, hanging between large pre-installed hooks, during trips that can last one or more weeks.

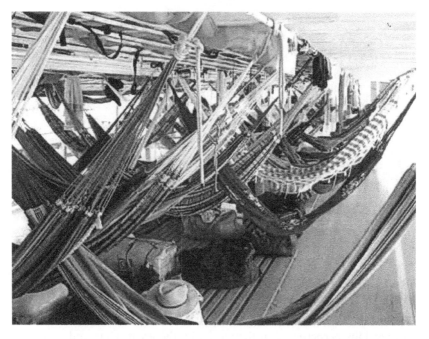

Figure 2.3 Colorful Brazilian hammocks are the most common sleeping places on board the riverboat *gaiolas* that criss-cross the Amazon River. In the absence of a network of roads, *gaiolas* are among the most popular ways to travel in Brazil's immense rainforest-covered north. These "river buses" connect small hamlets as well as large cities such as Belém and Manaus through trips that may last an entire week. Travelers bring their own hammocks and use the sturdy hooks available everywhere on deck. (Photo by Peter J. Kurz.)

Other descriptions speak of the search for an appropriate level of heat or cold. To write his important work about the Achuar tribe of Jivaros in the Upper Amazon jungles of Peru and Ecuador, the French anthropologist Philippe Descola lived for several years among this tribe with a reputation for "headhunting." He wrote in his classic, *The Spears of Twilight*:

> Unlike many other Amazonian tribes, the *Jivaros* use not hammocks but rectangular bedsteads covered by flexible slats of palm wood or bamboo . . . . You sleep in a strange position there, with your feet projecting into the void as they rest on a little bar set over a smouldering hearth. This arrangement is inspired by an old piece of popular lore according to which you never get cold so long as your feet are warm . . . The beds in the house are enclosed on three sides by wooden slats. In this dwelling without walls these offer a small island of privacy.

Unfortunately, the only bed available to him as a guest did not have this feature since it was "positioned alongside the outer roof supports, barely sheltered from the rain by the roof's overhang" and almost fully embedded in "the nocturnal echoes of the wildlife: a strident chorus produced by frogs and crickets and the throbbing bass of the toads . . . punctuated by the melancholy cries of predators and the three descending notes of the nightjar's whistle" (Descola 1993, 43).

Another centuries-old question has been: *Why sleep at night?* With the arrival of electricity (and computers), sleeping at night is very often neither chosen nor possible. But even before the effects of twentieth century shift work, soldiers and sailors stood night watches. And we can add the many well-documented cases of talented and productive individuals who preferred to sleep during the day. One of Hungary's literary giants, the great poet Sándor Weöres, declared at age 16 that he wished to sleep during the daylight hours and would study or work at night. He adhered to his chosen schedule for the rest of his long and productive life and made sleep and dreams one of his lifetime themes. Among his close friends was Árpád Illés, the equally talented and prolific abstract painter whose extraordinary egg tempera works of art continue to dazzle. One well-known Illés oil painting shows the 30-year-old Weöres sleeping midday in his small rural hometown of Csönge. From an early age he made it his habit to sleep during the day and write at night.

Many of the names and details of these myths changed through the centuries. Some can be attributed to the individual likes and preferences of succeeding narrators; others are due to differing versions created by different translators. They all have in common a universal appeal and are clear evidence of the perennial, continuing fascination of all humans with the relationship of sleep, dreams, and, at times, death. These stories and

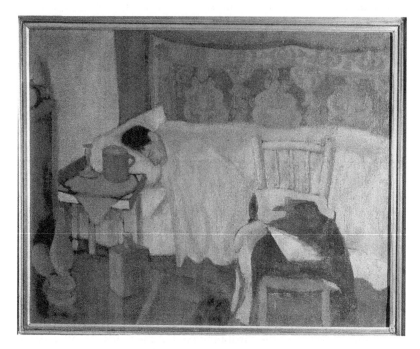

Figure 2.4 Hungarian poet Sándor Weöres asleep midday at age 30 in his rural hometown of Csönge. From an early age Weöres made it his habit to sleep during the day and write at night. This 1943 oil painting was done by his close friend Árpád. Over a period of almost half a century, Weöres, the poet, and Illés, the artist, collaborated in numerous joint literary and artistic projects, many of them focusing on the nature and essence of sleep and dreaming. Reproduction of *Weöreséknél Csöngén, Weöres Sándor alszik* (1943, canvas) by Árpád Illés (1908–1980). Photographer: Ádám Illés. Collection: Budapest/Hungary, Petőfi Irodalmi Múzeum. (Reprinted with permission from the Petőfi Literary Museum Fine Art Department, Budapest.)

myths are present from the earliest times and in all cultures, one way or another. They were attempts at explaining the relationship, for instance, between "sleep" and "death" through an imagined world based on real and universal experiences. Clearly both were part of all animal life and were different one from the other – but how? And why? The purpose here is to bring attention to this search for understanding, for answers, explanations, and to note that similar issues were (and are) even more present and more complex with the equally universal attempts at understanding the phenomenon we call hypnosis.

We can easily agree that a hypnotic state is not to death as Hypnos was to Thanatos. But less clear is the relationship of Hypnos and hypnosis – they seem to be similar, but are they related? If not, what is the difference and can it be demonstrated convincingly that they are two different states, "sleep" and a "hypnotic state"? If they are different, do they have clearly distinguishable characteristics and purposes?

There are many extraordinary works readily available (some listed in our references) which can provide the interested reader with a thorough understanding of our current state of knowledge. The purpose of this chapter and the next is to show how until now the flow of our understanding of the state of sleep has been based primarily on myths, legends, and descriptions or personal recollections through art, literature, and the words of philosophers; and that this started to change in a very significant and rapid way very recently – only a few decades ago. To a lesser extent, the same may be the case with hypnosis but, we believe, in a different manner, which will also be summarized in later chapters.

Everywhere, from the earliest days, our ancestors and those around them were curious and perplexed about the nature and meaning of sleep. They couldn't quite understand how or why it happened and, in many cultures, associated sleep with death. We have seen how the Greeks related the two through the myth of the brothers Sleep and Death (Hypnos and Thanatos) and their sisters, the three Keres. Another way was to believe that sleep was merely "a short death" in contrast with death, "a long sleep." Through a great variety of myths and fables our ancestors tried to understand and to explain the meaning of sleep. Many of these early attempts survived time and traveled from one region to another. For almost 18 centuries, the early Greek myths were replaced by the more "scientific" reasoning of Plato, Aristotle, and others who believed that the gases rising from our stomachs as food decomposed somehow affected the brain and caused periodic sleep. Other versions claimed that blood had a way of flooding the head and that such cyclical incoming and outgoing tides caused sleep.

Within the past century our understanding changed radically as new tools were developed and helped us see better, to analyze, study, and understand in a very different way. These tools give us our new ability to look inside the sleeping brain. Through the actual recording of electrical activity in the brain, scientists are now engaged in the emerging new science of sleep. We will show that many of the interpretations, depictions, and suppositions related to sleep that have been offered during the past millennia are not valid – that most were inaccurate. At the same time we will also try to show that in light of recent scientific findings we must marvel at the remarkable insights reflected in the works of many of these authors and artists.

What is Sleep? Moving Away from Myths and Fables

Now, as we turn our attention to how modern scientists view sleep we begin to learn more specific characteristics of this state beyond what was derived from careful but not scientific observations. One of the pioneers of sleep medicine has pointed out that "mostly, people describe sleep by saying what it is not." In *The Promise of Sleep*, Dement adds that "we say that sleeping is not being awake." When asked for a "simile for sleep," many cultures refer to "the ultimate switching off – death" or believe that "the soul leaves the body as we sleep and returns in the morning" (Dement and Vaughan 1999, 15).

Dement's own definition of sleep is anchored and defined in terms of "two essential features," as follows: "The first, and by far the most important, is that sleep erects a perceptual wall between the conscious mind and the outside world." He points out that this is not because of silence or closing off light. "The second defining feature of normal sleep is that it is immediately reversible." If immediate reversal cannot occur, "the person is not asleep, but unconscious or dead" (Dement and Vaughan 1999, 17). He also notes that coma, anesthesia, and hibernation, for instance, do not qualify as sleep for exactly this reason: from those states a person cannot be immediately aroused. Similarly, "since sleep cuts people off from most outside sounds, hypnosis – which allows its subjects to respond to suggestion – can't be considered sleep in any sense of the word." In addition to these key defining factors, Dement also lists important qualities of sleep (including that it occurs naturally – unlike anesthesia or hypnosis – and periodically). Finally, the significant big change in brain research: we now know that "sleep also is characterized by electrical changes in the brain, which scientists can measure using machines called electroencephalographs (EEGs), which graphically show brain waves" (Dement and Vaughan 1999, 17).

As a result of the scientific advances during the past hundred years, we now also know that light or the absence of light is not the cause of our need to sleep. We can, confidently, dismiss many other earlier, inaccurate suppositions. In his excellent *Power Sleep*, James B. Maas offers the following summary:

> We still need to sleep even though we have artificial illumination to counter darkness. Sleep doesn't occur in response to boredom or mental or physical fatigue. Sleep isn't necessary to conserve energy. Sleep is not determined by eating or by the resulting stomach vapors that Aristotle and the Greek philosophers thought cooled the heart or blocked the brain's pores. Nor is sleep determined by will. And sleep does not mean the cessation of brain activity – that happens only in animal hibernation.
>
> (Maas 1998, 26)

So, then, what is sleep? According to Maas:

> Rather than being a vast wasteland of monotonous inertness, sleep is a diverse, complex, multifaceted series of stages that make important contributions to our daytime functioning. The various stages

of sleep we experience each night as our senses disengage from the environment are delineated by significant changes in brain waves, muscle activity, eye movements, body temperature, respiration, heart rate, hormonal activity, and even genital arousal. The overall level of neural activity drops by only 10 percent during sleep. In fact, the "sleeping" brain is often significantly more active than the "awake" brain.

(Maas 1998, 27)

Far from just "resting," or being shut down or inactive, even while asleep the brain is surprisingly active:

We now know that various activities of the sleeping brain play a dramatic role in regulating gastrointestinal, cardiovascular, and immune functions, in energizing the body, and in cognitive processing, including the storing, reorganization, and eventual retrieval of information already in the brain, as well as in the acquisition of new information while awake.

(Maas 1998, 27)

In addition to attempts to define sleep, we have always tried to measure this mysterious, cyclical, and essential part of our lives. Recording and measuring the more obvious outward manifestations or episodes seen as associated with sleep, such as snoring or sleepwalking, was easy and is frequently reflected in art and literature.

"Sleep and Sleep Disorders in *Don Quixote*," by Iranzo, Santamaria, and de Riquer, is an insightful compilation of the numerous sleep-related vignettes that can be found in the Cervantes masterpiece. And, of course, other studies and analyses have shown that similar observations were made throughout recorded history. From the abstract:

Cervantes included masterful descriptions of several sleep disorders such as insomnia, sleep deprivation, disruptive loud snoring and rapid eye movement sleep behavior disorder. In addition, he described the occurrence of physiological, vivid dreams and habitual, post-prandial sleepiness – the siesta. Cervantes' concept of sleep as a passive state where all cerebral activities are almost absent is in conflict with his description of abnormal behaviours during sleep and vivid, fantastic dreams. His concept of sleep was shared by his contemporary, Shakespeare, and could have been influenced by the reading of the classical Spanish book of psychiatry *Examen de Ingenios* (1575)

(Iranzo, Santamaria, and de Riquer 2004, 97–100)

We know from experience that, regularly, one-third of our 24-hour day is devoted to sleep. Recording, measuring, comparing – they are all initial steps in our natural desire to learn more about how each average 70-year-old person today spends those 205,000+ hours or more than 8,500 24-hour days! How long did we sleep? How often was it interrupted? And why? How does that compare to the sleep of other mammals? Of other animals? Does one species sleep more frequently or adhere to a different cycle than another? Why are owls "night" owls? How could whales, dolphins, and fish sleep and swim? The answers that were recorded and survived through the ages were until recently limited to very basic facts which were further limited and, at times, distorted by the talents and limitations of the narrators and artists.

We do not need sophisticated technology to measure how long it takes for someone to fall asleep, or, if awakened during the night, to measure how long that person stayed awake before falling back asleep again. More difficult are the "why" questions: "Why do we need to sleep?" or "Why does one person sleep better and longer than another?" Even for a "normal" person who is "healthy" the follow-up questions are endless: What makes it easier or harder to sleep: light, noise, alcohol, hunger, heat, cold, the bed, or the pillow? Could it be related to "stress" or "worry"?

These are all questions that have been asked in the past, yet only recently can be answered more specifically. J. Allan Hobson is Emeritus Professor of Psychiatry, Harvard Medical School, and the author of numerous excellent books related to waking, sleeping, and dreaming. He considers "the decade between 1890 and 1900" to be the beginning of the time frame "in which the psychological and neurophysiological study of the brain/mind took on its current 'modern' form" (Hobson and Wohl 2005, 130).

He relates this beginning to the publication in 1890 of William James's *Principles of Psychology*, "which began with a chapter of what was then known about the brain and declared that brain science was fundamental to psychology in all of its aspects including the transcendent, the spiritual and the supernatural."

What is Sleep? New Tools and Technologies Help Us Begin to Understand

This is the beginning of the new science of the brain. It is difficult to overstate advances in our new understanding of the physiology of the human brain. The discovery of photography, then of "moving pictures," introduced the basic technology which was soon followed by the (accidental) invention of X-rays.

The recording of images through pinholes in a *camera obscura* was already known by the Greeks thousands of years ago. Black and white photography as we know it only began around 1832–1834, with the first color photographs arriving some 30 years later. Those discoveries and their increasingly popular introduction into everyday life began a rapid succession of further discoveries in imaging technology.

The discovery of X-rays in 1895 led to a revolutionary change in how scientists could see, record, and understand the human body. Wilhelm Conrad Roentgen (1845–1923) was the newly appointed Rector of the University of Würzburg when he developed the process which led to the first "photograph" of a person's human bones – a picture of his wife's hand that clearly showed the bones of her fingers, and the ring on her finger. A few weeks later *The New York Times* announced the discovery as a new form of photography that revealed hidden solids, penetrated wood, paper, and flesh, and exposed the bones of the human frame.

Our path to the modern tools that enable today's increased understanding of the brain – and, therefore, of sleep and hypnosis – continues with the many important contributions of Santiago Ramón y Cajal (1852–1934), the Spanish medical doctor and researcher who received the Nobel Prize in Physiology or Medicine in 1906.

Estimates of the number of neurones in the human brain vary, as does their function. The latest estimate today is that the human brain has approximately 86 billion neurones based on research isolating nuclei by Suzana Herculano-Houzel (presented at TEDGlobal 2013).

Entering the twentieth century, neurones were a bigger mystery than they are today. Ramón y Cajal's great contribution is fundamental to modern neuroscience. As summarized by Hobson:

> In its emphasis on the discreteness of neurones as the structural units of the brain, Cajal's work provided the paradigm that has guided neuroscience successfully for a century. Now that it is combined with the genetic model, it seems likely to continue to be germinal for at least another 100 years. Ramón y Cajal was much more than a journeyman anatomist. He was also a psychologist who, like Freud, was fascinated by the effects of hypnosis. Moreover, he was an accomplished draftsman who made all of the pen-and-ink renderings of neurones that illustrate his papers and books.
>
> (Hobson and Wohl 2005, 131)

Our "first insights" into the physiological mechanisms of sleep began with the discovery of the alpha wave in 1924, also known as "Berger's wave" after its discoverer, the German psychiatrist, physiologist, and neurologist Hans Berger (1873–1941). Berger developed and used for the first time the technology which revolutionized daily neurologic procedures: the EEG. Until the introduction of computed tomography in the 1970s, this was the principal instrument for recording brain waves. High-frequency and low-amplitude brain waves reflected a waking state, whereas low-frequency and high-amplitude brain waves were found to indicate a sleeping brain.

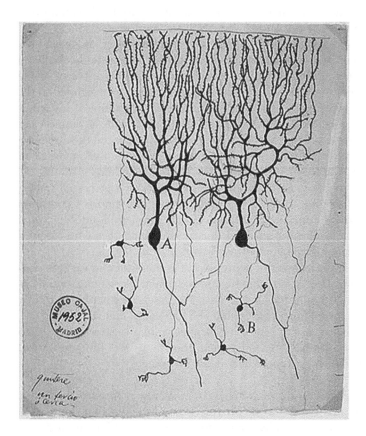

Figure 2.5 A drawing of the Purkinje cell by Santiago Ramón y Cajal,
the Spanish neuroanatomist who won the 1906 Nobel Prize in
Physiology or Medicine for his pioneering work on neurons. This
drawing of the Purkinje cell dendritic tree – a type found in the
cerebellum – is among his personal favorites. (Reproduced courtesy
of the Museo Cajal, Madrid [public domain].)

In 1925 the Russian-born sleep researcher Nathaniel Kleitman
(1895–1999) established at the University of Chicago the first laboratory
dedicated to the study of sleep. In 1939 he published his monumental
Sleep and Wakefulness, a 429-page compendium which "covered absolutely everything that was known about sleep up to 1939," according
to his future student and colleague, William C. Dement. In 1953 he
and his Chicago group discovered and described rapid eye movement
(REM) sleep.

Around 1948, two neurophysiologists, the American Horace Magoun
(1907–1991) and the Italian Giuseppe Moruzzi (1910–1986), collaborated in the study of the mechanisms underlying the control of
the sleep–waking cycle in mammals. Through the study of EEGs that

recorded electrical stimulation related to synchronized and desynchronized patterns, they identified the area of the brain responsible for maintaining wakefulness (the reticular activating system). Their studies and revelations are considered by many to have provided the basis for our ability to study the physiology of sleep. Walter Hess (1881–1973), a Swiss physiologist, discovered that there was a region in the brain (in the hypothalamus) which when stimulated in cats induced them to do the opposite – to sleep. He was awarded the 1949 Nobel Prize in Physiology or Medicine.

Rapid Eye Movement Sleep: The New Science of Sleep Emerges

Research on sleep reached a new level in 1952 when REMs during sleep were discovered, "essentially by accident in Nathaniel Kleitman's lab" at the University of Chicago (Lockley and Foster 2012, 6). Kleitman and his students in the Chicago lab studied many aspects of sleep, including, of course, the close observation of eye movements during sleep, a study conducted with his Ph.D. student, Eugene Aserinsky (1921–1998). During this time Dement, also a pioneer in sleep research, had arrived in Chicago to begin his studies at the medical school in September, 1951. In *The Promise of Sleep*, Dement describes in a fascinating, entertaining, and informative style those well-known and now classic experiments which introduced the age of our new science of sleep (Dement and Vaughan 1999). According to Dement, a lecture by Kleitman so motivated him that he volunteered for work in his sleep laboratory. Upon acceptance he was directed to "help Gene Aserinsky, who is trying to record eye movements during sleep." Aserinsky was a graduate student in physiology who had been given the assignment to observe rolling eye movements during sleep, to see if they might be an indicator of "the depth of sleep." Aserinsky had begun his study of the slow eye movements the year before, in 1951. According to Maas:

> He detected these rolling movements by observing the shifting bulges of the cornea under sleeping infants' thin eyelids. In the course of his observations Aserinsky made a remarkable discovery. At various times during sleep the infants' eyes vigorously darted back and forth, up and down. These rapid eye movements appeared to be similar to those observed in the waking stage.
>
> (Maas 1998, 28)

To find a more complete answer to the many related questions – Were these merely an indicator of sleep, or muscle twitches? Were the infants dreaming? – an experiment was devised in 1952 that relied on the use of the EEG. Aserisky, Kleitman, and Dement "attached a pair of small recording electrodes to the faces of adult volunteers, near the outside corners of their eyes" and with the help of an EEG machine collected records of the electrical signals (Maas 1998, 28).

The principles of electromagnetism have been known since the late eighteenth century and by the mid nineteenth century it was also known that small currents produced by living tissue could be recorded. Yet the 1952–1953 breakthroughs occurred partly because the EEG used for the experiments in Kleitman's laboratory was a "junked" device "resurrrected" by Aserinsky that kept malfunctioning (Alvarez 1995, 94).[5]

In one of his experiments, Aserinsky connected the EEG to his sleeping eight-year-old son's eyes. "But the broken-down machine went on breaking down, no matter how often Aserinsky fixed it," according to an account in *Night*. "Even when it seemed to be running properly, recording the slow waves of the boy's rolling eye movements, its pens intermittently went wild, tracing jagged peaks and troughs similar to those of the waking brain." When he kept getting the same "improbable results" he realized "that he might have stumbled on a significant discovery" (Alvarez 1995, 90).

As noted by Dement:

> I believe that the study of sleep became a true scientific field in 1953, when I finally was able to make all-night, continuous recordings of brain and eye activity during sleep. The most profound point to make is that for the first time, it was possible to carry out continuous observations of sleep without disturbing the sleeper. In addition, science is largely quantification, and this work was the beginning of studying sleep as a whole for its own sake and of describing and quantifying its overall patterns through the night.
>
> (Dement and Vaughn 1999, 38)[6]

According to Dement, these all-night recordings resulted in three major observations. First, that the periodic REMs were "part of a 90-minute basic sleep cycle" and "a major discovery" that "everybody, without exception, had the same pattern of sleep" (Dement and Vaughan 1999). Second, that there were five distinct stages of sleep. And third, that REM movements only occurred in the final, fifth stage, which he then called REM sleep.

In his thoroughly enjoyable first-person account of these significant discoveries, Dement adds the following vignette: "at the time, I made up these names casually, having no idea that the same names would still be used almost 50 years later" and "simply making up the names for sleep stages is something I would never have the audacity to do now" (Dement and Vaughan 1999).

These discoveries encouraged Dement to immerse himself in the observation of REM sleep in the most diverse groups of people he could find, healthy as well as sick, of different ages and backgrounds, including infants.

He also recounts that in the 1950s women were not participants in all-night sleep studies yet, despite this opposition (apparently based on fear of "scandal for either the laboratory" or its researchers), Dement received restricted permission from Kleitman to conduct the "chaperoned" study that is now considered to have been the first overnight sleep study on a woman (Dement and Vaughan 1999).[7]

Since 1953, the study of sleep and sleep medicine has changed rapidly. In 1970 Dement founded the world's first sleep disorder center at Stanford University, where he has continued his pioneering and groundbreaking research. The first issue of the journal *Sleep* was published in 1978. In 1981, a revolutionized treatment of sleep apnea was introduced through the use of nasal continuous positive airway pressure (CPAP) machines. In Minnesota, a group led by Carlos Schenck and Mark Mahowald first described REM sleep behavior disorder in 1986. All this promises to be a mere beginning, with further advances expected through the constant improvement of existing tools, the introduction of new techniques (functional magnetic resonance imaging (fMRI), nuclear MRI) and remarkable findings through amazing research.

As summarized in *The Promise of Sleep*:

> What used to be rough speculation by natural philosophers now has become a solid science wherein we can record electrical brain waves and characterize them across the spectrum of consciousness and unconsciousness, from full alertness to drowsiness, through all the stages of sleep and dreaming.
>
> (Dement and Vaughan 1999)

The Science of Sleep

Sleep is more than the absence of wakefulness. It serves numerous vital functions for the optimal homeostasis of the individual. Berger's recordings of the brain waves of humans in 1924 resulted in a method of evaluating the function of the central nervous system and researchers thereafter began to look for changes occurring inside the cranium. Since that time, rapid progress has been made in our understanding of the underlying physiology and neurochemistry of sleep. With the development of polysomnography in the 1950s and 1960s a way of measuring sleep was established. Efforts began to catalog the measurement of sleep in a more standardized manner and in 2007 and 2014 these were updated through revised editions of the *Manual for the Scoring of Sleep and Associated Events* under the auspices of the American Academy of Sleep Medicine (AASM). (A brief review of recent developments in the treatment of sleep disorders will be discussed in Chapter 7.)

Sleep architecture as currently defined is based on the consensus of sleep experts in the AASM *Manual for the Scoring of Sleep and Associated*

Events (AASM 2014). Sleep is broken down into non-REM (NREM) and REM states, in addition to the waking state, comprising three distinctive states of existence. Sleep architecture is based on changes in the EEG, electrooculogram (EOG), and electromyogram (EMG). The EEG records differences in electrical potential generated by the apical dendrites of cortical neurons using scalp electrodes. The EOG records eye movements based on electrical differences between the anterior and posterior chamber of the eye, with the aqueous humor being positive and the vitreous negative in polarity. The EMG records electrical muscle tension. These three parameters (EMG, EOG, EEG) are utilized to define the various stages of sleep. Additional measures are utilized in clinical evaluation, including electrocardiogram, airflow, chest and abdominal movement, and leg movements. EEG frequencies include alpha (8–12 Hz), theta (4–7 Hz), delta (0.5–3 Hz), beta (14–30 Hz), and gamma (30–50 Hz centered on 40 Hz). For the purpose of scoring sleep stages, sleep is broken into 30-second epochs.

In the future, other modalities may more accurately describe the neural changes occurring during sleep and yield more specific information that would be helpful clinically.

Based on the above electrophysiological events, sleep has been divided into REM and NREM sleep.

REM sleep is characterized by relatively low-voltage mix frequency EEG pattern, with REMs and relatively low EMG muscle tone.

REM is probably controlled by cholinergic brainstem mechanisms in the pontine brainstem. Wakefulness and REM sleep share common EEG properties. Elevated brain activity is present during REM as well as during the waking state, causing the term paradoxical sleep to be applied to REM. REM sleep has been linked to vivid dreaming. Oxygen consumption is increased during REM and there is irregularity of heart rate and breathing. Body temperature is not well regulated (poikilothermia). Skeletal muscles are paralyzed in REM secondary to motor neurone inhibition. Penile erection normally accompanies REM sleep, as does erection of the clitoris.

REM sleep can be divided into tonic REM and phasic REM, although clinically this is not usually done. Phasic REM is sympathetically driven and is characterized by REMs, muscle twitches, and respiratory variability. Tonic REM is parasympathetically driven and is characterized by low EMG tone. Takahara, Nittono, and Hori (2002) compared event-related potentials during wakefulness and REM using an auditory discrimination task. REM sleep was separated into phasic REM and tonic REM. They found that the brain was less sensitive to external stimuli during phasic REM than during tonic REM. Wehrle et al. (2007), utilizing fMRI on 11 subjects, studied the difference in function of tonic and phasic REM by applying acoustic stimulation. They found that during tonic REM acoustic stimulation elicited a residual activation of the auditory cortex; however, during phasic REM there appeared to be a lack of reactivity to sensory stimuli.

NREM sleep is broken down into three stages: N1, N2, and N3. Stage N1 consists of low-voltage mixed-frequency background EEG with cessation of blinking in the absence of saccadic eye movements and less than 50% alpha activity.

Stage N2 is defined by bursts of 14–16-Hz wave sleep spindles, and high-amplitude short-duration K complexes with less than 20% of the epoch in slow-wave sleep (SWS).

Stage N3 is defined by the presence of high-voltage slow delta waves comprising more than 20% of the epoch.

The waking-state EEG activity consists of low-voltage fast waves with the patient alert. With the eyes closed and the patient relaxed, a predominant alpha pattern is generated.

The sleep pattern across the night varies with age. Characteristic patterns of sleep architecture change throughout the developmental process. Everyone has their own variation of this developmental sleep pattern.

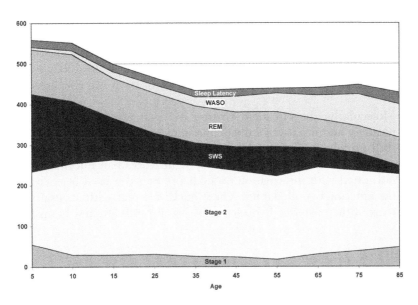

Figure 2.6 Age-related trends for sleep stage 1, stage 2 sleep, slow-wave sleep (SWS), rapid eye movement (REM) sleep, wake after sleep onset (WASO), and sleep latency (in minutes). (Reproduced with permission from Ohayon, Maurice M., Mary A. Carskadon, Christian Guilleminault, and Michael V. Vitiello. 2004. "Meta-Analysis of Quantitative Sleep Parameters From Childhood to Old Age in Healthy Individuals: Developing Normative Sleep Values Across the Human Lifespan." *Sleep*, Vol 27, Issue 7: 1255–1273, © 2004. Permission conveyed through Copyright Clearance Center, Inc.)

Typically the young adult spends 20–25% in REM stage, 50% in stage N2, 12.5–20% in stage N3 and the remainder in stage N1. The newborn spends almost 50% of sleep time in REM stage, and this gradually decreases with age. REM sleep plateaus in childhood and is maintained well into old age. The newborn enters sleep through REM stage whereas older infants and adults enter sleep through stage N1. Sleep cycles occur throughout the night in approximately 90-minute episodes for adults, with the first REM occurring approximately 90 minutes after going to sleep. The first REM period is relatively short and increases during subsequent episodes. Most of the SWS is in the first third of the night and most REM in the last third.

Just as there are significant individual differences in the need for the amount of total sleep, the amount of time in each stage varies by individual with a probable genomic component.

Sleep is regulated by neural systems within the brain. There are two main processes: process C, the circadian rhythm, and process S, the homeostatic drive. Process C is regulated by the suprachiasmatic nucleus located in the anterior hypothalamus. Process S is determined by the amount of time that has lapsed since the last episode of sleep with the accumulation of neurotransmitters such as adenosine and promoted by neurones in the ventral lateral pre-optic area.

Despite curiosity concerning the role of sleep, until recently very little knowledge about the function of sleep was available. In 2002, Pace-Schott and Hobson reviewed the neurobiology of sleep and concluded:

> Molecularly, the circadian rhythm of sleep involves interlocking positive- and negative-feedback mechanisms of circadian genes and their protein products in cells of the suprachiasmatic nucleus that are entrained to ambient conditions by light. Circadian information is integrated with information on homeostatic sleep need in nuclei of the anterior hypothalamus. These nuclei interact with arousal systems in the posterior hypothalamus, basal forebrain and brainstem

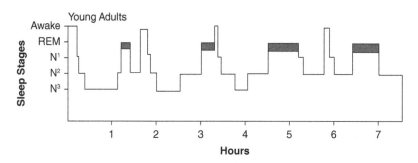

Figure 2.7 Hypnogram of young adult sleep. REM, rapid eye movement.

to control sleep onset. During sleep, an ultradian oscillator in the mesopontine junction controls the regular alteration of rapid eye movement (REM) and non-REM sleep. Sleep cycles are accompanied by neuromodulatory influences on forebrain structures that influence behavior, consciousness, and cognition.

(Pace-Schott and Hobson 2002, 591)

A good review of the neurophysiological mechanisms of sleep and wakefulness can be found in *Seminars in Neurology* (2004), by Sinton and McCarley. In spite of the recent developments in sleep research, the ultimate meaning or need for sleep remains controversial. Based on current knowledge, the purpose of sleep remains largely theoretical. When evaluating sleep function along with the consequences of insufficient sleep, differences between associated, contributing, and causal relationships need to be kept in mind.

Sleep is not only a global process but regional changes within the brain occur during sleep. Werth, Achermann, and Borbely, utilizing EEG spectral analysis compared changes occurring along the anterior–posterior axis in NREM and REM sleep. They concluded "that the neuronal processes underlying the sleep EEG differ between brain regions and support the notion that sleep is a local, use-dependent phenomenon" (Werth, Achermann, and Borbely 1997, 111).

Sleep appears necessary for optimum physical, psychological, and cognitive function. Sleep loss has been associated with irritability, depression, and tiredness. Impaired memory and cognitive dysfunction increase with sleep loss. With severe sleep loss, hallucinatory activity may occur. Deterioration in neurobehavioral function accumulates across days of partial sleep loss to levels similar to those found after total sleep loss of one to three nights. Poor decision making secondary to sleep loss has been reported to be involved in serious accidents such as Chernobyl, Three Mile Island, and the Challenger disaster. Sleep loss is rapidly becoming the number one cause of carnage on the highways.

There is significant individual variability as to the number of hours needed for each individual to maintain optimum functioning. Typically adults need seven to eight hours of sleep. Getting too little sleep or too much sleep can have adverse health effects. Changes in metabolic and endocrine function along with changes in immune and inflammatory responses have been shown to occur with sleep restriction. Sleep loss affects emotional, declarative, and procedural memory.

In 1972 I collaborated with Drs. Ismet Karacan and Owen Rennert (Kohler, Karacan, and Rennert, 1972) in evaluating a circadian pattern for RNA synthesis in human leukocytes. Total RNA was evaluated along with 4S and 5S RNA. A definite circadian pattern was present, with the 4S curve having a significant inverse relationship to the 5S curve. The possibility of an anabolic function for sleep was raised.

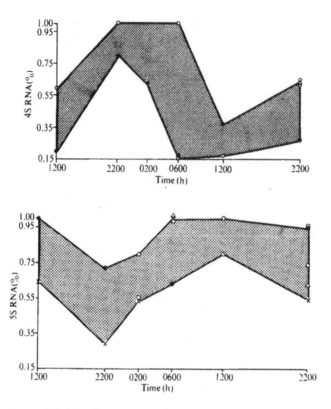

Figure 2.8 Circadian pattern of RNA synthesis. (Reproduced with
permission from Kohler, William C., Ismet Karacan, and Owen
M. Rennert. 1972. "Circadian Variation of RNA in Human
Leucocytes." *Nature* 238 (5359) (July 14):94–96.)

Bennington and Heller (1995) presented a model of sleep function in
which NREM sleep is essential for replenishment of cerebral glycogen
stores which are depleted during awakening. Maquet et al. (1990), utilizing positron emission tomography (PET), evaluated cerebral glucose
utilization during sleep and wakefulness. They found that during REM
sleep cerebral glucose utilization was similar to that of wakefulness. The
rate of glucose utilization in SWS was significantly lower than that of
wakefulness. They hypothesized that "energy requirements for maintaining membrane polarity are reduced during SWS because of a decreased
rate of synaptic events" (Maquet et al. 1990, 136).

Sleep is involved in the regulation of glucose homeostasis and various
hormonal regulations. Hormonal production may adhere to a circadian
or ultradian rhythm, whereas in the case of growth hormone, it is related

to SWS. The role of sleep in metabolic function is reviewed by Morselli, Guyon, and Spiegel (2012).

Sleep also serves an important role in immune function. Chronic sleep loss creates an inflammatory response. Faraut et al. (2012) reported increases in neutrophil counts after sleep restriction. A nap after eight hours of sleep, or ten hours of recovery sleep, returned values to near baseline. Imeri and Opp (2009) reviewed the relationship between the immune system and sleep. They pointed out that changes in sleep architecture occurred during infection. REM sleep is suppressed and NREM sleep is increased but is more fragmented. Fever is important to survival from infections.

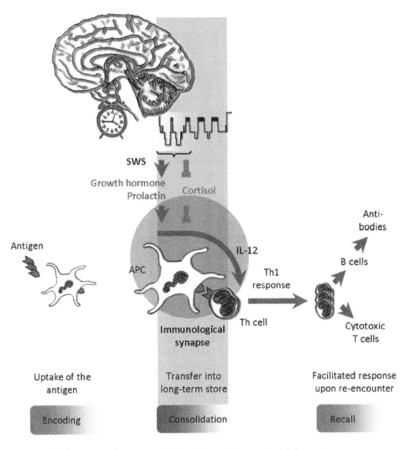

Figure 2.9 Immune function during sleep. (Reproduced from Luciana Besedovsky, Tanja Lange, and Jan Born. 2012. "Sleep and Immune Function." *Pflugers Archiv – European Journal of Physiology* Volume 463: 121–137, with kind permission from Springer Science + Business Media.)

In REM sleep we are essentially poikilothermic without response to temperature variations with shivering or sweating. Besedovsky, Lange, and Born (2012) review immune function and sleep.

Xie et al. evaluated the role of natural sleep or anesthesia in live mice using real-time assessments of tetramethylammonium diffusion and 2-photon imaging. They found that:

> natural sleep or anesthesia are associated with a 60% increase in the interstitial space, resulting in a striking increase in convective exchange of cerebral spinal fluid with interstitial fluid. In turn convective fluxes of interstitial fluid increased the rate of (beta) amyloid clearance during sleep. Thus, the restorative function of sleep may be a consequence of the enhanced removal of potentially neurotoxic waste products that accumulate in the awake central nervous system.
>
> (Xie et al. 2013, 373)

This study gives evidence that potentially one of the main purposes of sleep is the removal of toxic metabolic byproducts from the brain. Toxic wastes are flushed out of the brain into the blood stream and then to the liver for detoxification. (Beta)amyloids and A(beta)oligomers, which are degradation products of cellular activity, are cleared during sleep. If these are not removed, synaptic transmission is negatively affected. Lack of sleep hinders this process.

One of the more intriguing hypotheses pertaining to the need for sleep is associated with cognitive function and memory consolidation. Memory encoding and retrieval take place during waking whereas consolidation of memory occurs during sleep. In their 2010 review of memory function of sleep, Diekelmann and Born concluded that:

> SWS sleep and REM sleep have complementary functions to optimize memory consolidation. During slow wave sleep, characterized by slow oscillation-induced widespread synchronization of neuronal activity, active system consolidation integrates newly encoded memories with pre-existing long-term memories, thereby inducing conformational changes in the respective representations.
>
> (Diekelmann and Born 2010, 123; a brief but good review of the neurotransmitters involved in sleep is present in their review on page 122, box 3)

The role of REM sleep appears to be particularly important in the development of procedural memory, which refers to memory for skills that are developed by repeated practice and may not be available to conscious recollection. Procedural memory relies on the striatum and cerebellum, as well as the hippocampus.

NREM sleep has recently been noted to be important for declarative memory. Declarative memory refers to memories that are accessible through conscious recollection. It is mediated by the hippocampal memory system and includes retention for facts and events. Memory, after initial encoding, is fragile and has to be reinforced to become permanent. Sleep has a role in supporting this consolidation.

There is an overlap in brain systems involved in memory, daytime somnolence, and hypnosis. The default mode network (DMN) is one particular example. The DMN is active during internally focused tasks such as autobiographical memory retrieval, and envisioning the future when the individual is not focused on the external environment. Hypnosis is associated with reduced activity in the DMN. Buckner et al. (2008) felt that there was a "possible adaptive role of the default network for using past experiences to plan for the future, navigate social interactions, and maximize utility of movements while we are not otherwise engaged by the external world." Ward et al. (2013) studied the relationship between chronic daytime somnolence and connectivity in six brain networks, including the DMN using fMRI. Only the DMN was correlated with daytime sleepiness. The Epworth Sleepiness Scale (ESS) was used to evaluate excessive daytime somnolence in 27 young adults and 84 elderly people. The researchers concluded that "daytime sleepiness is associated with impaired connectivity of the DMN in a manner that is distinct from the effects of aging" (Ward et al. 2013, 1609). Increasing ESS was related to decreasing DMN functional connectivity. There was no association between the ESS and functional connectivity in the primary sensory networks of the brain. Greicius et al. (2009) had previously shown that resting-state functional connectivity reflects structural connectivity in the DMN.

Sterpenich et al. studied the role of sleep in emotional memory consolidation in healthy volunteers utilizing fMRI, a technology that measures brain activity by detecting changes in blood flow. The volunteers were engaged in a recognition test 72 hours after exposure to neutral and emotional pictures and again at six months. One half had been totally sleep-deprived on the first encoding night, whereas the other half were allowed to sleep. After retesting at six months, subjects were asked to recall previously studied information and in addition were presented with new pictures. This revealed significantly larger responses in the non-sleep-deprived in the ventral medial prefrontal cortex and the precuneus, two areas of the brain which are involved in memory encoding. The study concluded that "sleep during the first post-encoding night profoundly influences the long-term systems-level consolidation of emotional memory and modifies the functional segregation and integration associated with recollection in the long-term" (Sterpenich et al. 2009, 5143). They felt that their findings concerning memory processing were more compatible with the hypothesis of Maquet (2001) than that of Tononi and Cirelli (2003). Maquet had proposed "a coordinated replay of the neural pattern between hippocampal and neocortical areas during sleep leading to the gradual memory storage within distributed cortical networks." Tononi and Cirelli had hypothesized that:

> learning would result in a net increase in synaptic strength in many brain circuits, a condition that is not energetically sustainable in the long term. The role of sleep, especially of the cellular activity associated with slow waves, would be a down-scale synaptic strength to a baseline level, a mechanism that would eventually consolidate memory
> (Sterpenich et al. 2009, 5151)

Gais et al. (2002) evaluated each stage of sleep, spindle density, and EEG power spectra after extensive training on a declarative learning task as compared to a non-learning control task of equal visual stimulation. During N2 sleep the spindle density was significantly higher after the learning condition than after the non-learning condition. They concluded that their findings indicated "spindle activity during non-REM sleep is sensitive to previous learning experience" (Gais et al. 2002, 6830). In 2007 Gais et al. reported changes in brain activity, utilizing fMRI, during recall of previously learned verbal material when subjects slept or were sleep-deprived on the first night after learning. They found that learning was improved with sleep. Functional connectivity between the hippocampus and the medial prefrontal cortex was enhanced.

Huber et al. (2004) asked subjects to perform a motor learning task just before going to sleep. Utilizing EEG spectral analysis Huber found that slow-wave activity was increased in the right parietal areas and that this local increase in SWS after learning correlated with improved task performance after sleep.

Lu and Göder (2012) reviewed the role of NREM sleep and declarative memory consolidation. NREM sleep has been felt to play a role in physiological functional restoration. More recently, a role in memory consolidation has been proposed. It has been suggested that declarative memories, which are accessible through conscious recollection, may also occur in sleep during the NREM stage, as noted previously. Lu and Göder reviewed studies in patients with schizophrenia, Alzheimer's disease, and fibromyalgia syndrome and concluded that abnormal EEG activity during NREM sleep was associated with declarative memory impairment. Declarative memory consolidation appeared to be disrupted with reduced SWS and reduced spindle activity.

A major step in understanding how sleep helps memory and learning was reported by Yang at al. (2014). By making small holes in the skulls of mice they were able to utilize microscopic imaging to evaluate changes in dendritic spines during sleep. They evaluated changes in the postsynaptic dendritic spines of the primary motor cortex in mice caused by motor learning. New spines were formed on different sets of dendritic branches in response to different learning tasks. If the mice were sleep-deprived there was a markedly decreased number of new spines. Sleep did not appear to have any effect on the rate of spine elimination.

The purpose of REM sleep is even more enigmatic. It comprises more than 40% of sleep in the newborn, which decreases with age, and has been shown to be associated with procedural memory encoding. Horne reviewed the potential role of REM sleep and concluded it "is more likely to prepare for ensuing wakefulness rather than provide recovery from prior wakefulness, as happens with 'deeper' nonREM. Many of REM's characteristics are 'wake-like' (unlike nonREM)" (Horne 2013, 152).

Sleep is more than the opposite of wakefulness; it performs a vital contribution to optimum functioning.

Notes

1 The writings of Miguel de Cervantes have been admired, praised, and enjoyed for innumerable obvious as well as very subtle reasons. Among the best-known quotes from *Don Quixote* and, perhaps, the most perceptive about the perennial questions humans have about sleep can be found in a dialogue between Don Quixote and his squire, Sancho Panza:

> No entiendo esto, replicó Sancho; solo entiendo que en tanto que duermo, ni tengo temor, ni esperanza, ni trabajo, ni gloria; y bien haya el que inventó el sueño, capa que cubre todos los humanos pensamientos, manjar que quita la hambre, agua que ahuyenta la sed, fuego que calienta el frío, frío que temple el ardor, y, finalmente, moneda general con que todas las cosas se compran, balanza y peso que iguala al pastor con el rey y al simple con el discreto. Sola una cosa tiene mala el sueño, según he oído deir, y es que se parece a la muerte, pues de un dormido a un muerto hay muy poca diferencia."
> (Cervantes, 2010, *Don Quixote*, Part II, Chapter LXVIII)

This famous dialogue by Cervantes is only one of many such references, observations, and wise insights into the worlds of sleep and dreaming.

2 "sueño, m." *Oxford Spanish Dictionary*. 2003. New York: Oxford University Press.

The first meaning of the word (A.1 on page 780) is given as "sleep"; the second (B.1, also on page 780) as "dream." There are other languages where the word for sleep and dream is either exactly the same or very closely related. Two examples are Hungarian and Catalan. The *magyar* word for both "dream" and "sleep" is *álom*.

3 The authors have not consulted or reviewed the following, earlier sources. They are provided here for the information of readers interested in additional details: Metaphrastes' version is in P. G., CXV, 427–448; Gregory of Tours, Passio VII Dormientium in the Anal. Bolland., XII, 371–387; Chardry, Li Set Dormanz, ed. Koch (Leipzig, 1879); Legenda Aurea and Caxton's version for July; Koch, Die Siebenschlafereigende, ihr Ursprung u. ihre Verbreitung (Leipzig, 1883); an exhaustive monograph with a full bibliography

4 In the original Spanish:

> Ahora bien, tornémonos a acomodar, y durmamos lo poco que queda de la noche, y amanecerá Dios y medraremos.

—Duerme tú, Sancho – respondió don Quijote –, que naciste para dormir; que yo, que nací para velar, en el tiempo que falta de aquí al día daré rienda a mis pensamientos, y los desfogaré en un madrigalete, que sin que tú lo sepas anoche compuse en la memoria.

—A mí me parece – respondió Sancho – que los pensamientos que dan lugar a hacer coplas no deben de ser muchos. Vuesa merced coplee cuanto qusiere, que yo dormiré cuanto pudiere.

5 Alvarez, A. *Night: Night Life, Night Language, Sleep and Dreams*. New York: W.W. Norton.

This highly informative as well as entertaining work is filled with insights and anecdotes, many collected during personal interviews. One example from his "introduction" of Eugene Aserinsky (p. 90):

The breakthrough was made by Eugene Aserinsky, a graduate student who had never graduated, a drop-out avant la lettre; he had dropped out of college without a degree, served in the Army, dropped out of dental school and dropped out of social work before he found his way to the University of Chicago, where he was taken in – "like a stray cat," he has said – by Nathaniel Kleitman, one of the founders of sleep research.

6 Dement, William C. and Christopher Vaughan. 1999. *The Promise of Sleep*. New York: Delacorte Press, Random House, 38.

On page 30 of this same chapter, Dr. Dement provides a good summary of his evaluation of the technological sciences that made possible the rapid advances in sleep medicine in the past century:

What I regard as the watershed series of technological advances that were necessary for the dawn of sleep science were, first, the discovery of spontaneous electrical activity in the brains of animals by Richard Coton in 1875, and next the demonstration by German psychiatrist Hans Berger in the late 1920s and early 1930s that the brains of human beings also showed spontaneous electrical activity that could be recorded from the scalp. Given the trials and tribulations I had in the early days with Kleitman trying to get decent brain wave recordings, I believe that Berger's demonstration with the primitive equipment available to him was nothing short of miraculous. He clearly identified the waking alpha rhythm and said that if a subject fell asleep, the rhythm disappeared and electrical activity was very low amplitude or sparse during sleep.

7 Dement, William C. and Christopher Vaughan. 1999. *The Promise of Sleep*. New York: Delacorte Press, Random House.

The following paragraph (from p. 40) adds yet another personal note related to this topic:

I obtained my M.D. in 1955, and while all my classmates went on to their internships I stayed behind to begin a $3,000-a-year research fellowship. Shortly thereafter I met Pat Weber, the woman who would later become my wife. She volunteered to be recorded on 20 consecutive nights to see if sleep patterns were the same every night in a single individual. It isn't true, however, that I married her to get a cooperative subject . . . .

As I continued to include an occasional woman in my sleep studies, there were always people who thought something untoward was going on.

References

Alvarez, A. 1995. *Night: Night Live, Night Language, Sleep and Dreams*. New York: W. W. Norton.

American Academy of Sleep Medicine (AASM) 2007. *Manual for the Scoring of Sleep and Associated Events: Rules, Terminology and Technical Specifications*. Darien, Il: American Academy of Sleep Medicine.

American Academy of Sleep Medicine (AASM). 2014. *Manual for the Scoring of Sleep and Associated Events: Rules, Terminology and Technical Specifications*. Version 2.1. Darien, Il: American Academy of Sleep Medicine.

Bennington, Joel H., and H. Craig Heller. 1995. "Restoration of Brain Energy Metabolism as the Function of Sleep." *Progress in Neurobiology* 45: 347–360.

Besedovsky, Luciana, Tanja Lange, and Jan Born. 2012. "Sleep and Immune Function." *Pflugers Archives – European Journal of Physiology* 463: 121–137.

Buckner, R. L., J. R. Andrews-Hanna, and D. L. Schacter. 2008. "The Brain's Default Network: Anatomy, Function, and Relevance to Disease." *Annals of the New York Academy of Science* 1124 (March): 1–38.

Cervantes, Miguel de. 2003. *Don Quixote (The Ingenious Gentleman Don Quixote of La Mancha)*. Translated by John Ormsby. Toronto: Penguin Classics.

Cervantes, Miguel de. 2010. *Don Quijote de la Mancha*. Madrid: Edimat Libros.

Dement, William C. and Christopher Vaughan. 1999. *The Promise of Sleep*. New York: Delacorte Press, Random House.

Descola, Philippe. 1993. *The Spears of Twilight. Life and Death in the Amazon Jungle*. Translated by Janet Lloyd. New York: New Press.

Diekelmann, Suzanne and Jan Born. 2010. "The Memory Function of Sleep." *Nature Reviews* 11 (February): 114–126.

Faraut, Brice, K. Z. Boudjeltia, L. Vanhamme, and M. Kerkhofs. 2012. "Immune Inflammatory and Cardiovascular Consequences of Sleep Restriction and Recovery." *Sleep Medicine Reviews* 16: 137–149.

Fortescue, Adrian. 1909. "The Seven Sleepers of Ephesus." In *The Catholic Encyclopedia*, Vol 5. New York: Appleton.

Gais, Steffan, Genevieve Albouy, Melanie Boly, Thien Thanh Dang-Vu, Annabelle Darsaud, Martin Desseilles, Geraldine Rauchs, Manuel Schabus, Virginie Sterpenich, Gilles Vandenwalle, Pierre Maquet, and Philippe Peigneux. 2007. "Sleep Transforms the Cerebral Trace of Declarative Memories." *Proceedings of the National Academy of Sciences of the United States of America* 104 (47): 18778–18783.

Gais, Steffan, Matthias Molie, Kay Helms, and Jan Born. 2002. "Learning-Dependent Increases in Sleep Spindle Density." *Journal of Neuroscience* 22 (15) (August 1): 6830–6834.

Greicius, Michael D., Kaustubh Supekar, Vinod Menon, and Robert F. Dougherty. 2009. "Resting-State Functional Connectivity Reflects Structural Connectivity in the Default Mode Network." *Cerebral Cortex* 19 (1) (January): 72–78.

Herculano-Houzel, Suzana. 2013. "Lessons From Brain Soup." *TEDglobal presentation*.

Hobson, J. Allan and Hellmut Wohl. 2005. *From Angels To Neurones: Art and The New Science of Dreaming*. Special Edition. Fidenza: Mattioli 1885.

Horne, Jim. 2013. "Why REM Sleep? Clues Beyond the Laboratory in a More Challenging World." *Biological Psychology* 92: 152–168.

Huber, Reto, M. Felice Ghlardi, Marcello Massimini, and Giulio Tononi. 2004. "Local Sleep and Learning." *Nature* 430 (July 1): 78–81.

Imeri, Luca and Mark R. Opp. 2009. "How (and Why) the Immune System Makes Us Sleep." *Nature Reviews/Neuroscience* 10 (March): 199–210.

Iranzo, Alex, Joan Santamaria, and Martin de Riquer. 2004. "Sleep and Sleep Disorders in *Don Quixote.*" *Journal of Sleep Medicine* 5 (1) (January): 97–100.

Kleitman, Nathaniel. 1939. *Sleep and Wakefulness.* Chicago, Il: University of Chicago Press: Midway Reprint. Revised edition April 1963.

Kohler, William C., Ismet Karacan, and Owen M. Rennert. 1972. "Circadian Variation of RNA in Human Leucocytes." *Nature* 238 (5359) (July 14): 94–96.

Lockley, Steven W. and Russell G. Foster. 2012. *Sleep: A Very Short Introduction.* Oxford: Oxford University Press.

Lu, William and Robert Göder. 2012. "Does Abnormal Non-Rapid Eye Movement Sleep Impair Declarative Memory Consolidation? Disturbed Thalamic Functions in Sleep." *Sleep Medicine Reviews* 16: 389–394.

Maas, James B. 1998. *Power Sleep: The Revolutionary Program That Prepares Your Mind for Peak Performance.* New York: Harper-Collins.

Maquet, Pierre. 2001. "The Role of Sleep in Learning and Memory." *Science* 294(1): 1048–1052.

Maquet, Pierre, Dominique Dive, Eric Salmon, Bernard Sadzot, Gianni Franco, Robert Poirrier, Remy von Frenckell, and Georges Franck. 1990. "Cerebral Glucose Utilization During Sleep–Wake Cycle in Man Determined by Positron Emission Tomography and [F]2-fluoro-2-deoxy-D-glucose Method." *Brain Research* 513: 136–143.

Morselli, Lisa L., Aurore Guyon, and Karine Spiegel. 2012. "Sleep and Metabolic Function." *Pflugers Archives – European Journal of Physiology* 463: 139–160.

Ormsby, John, trans. 2011. *The History of Don Quixote,* Vol. II. Ithaca, NY: Cornell University Library Digital Collections.

Oxford English Dictionary. 2014. New York: Oxford University Press. "sleep, n." *OED Online.* http://www.oed.com/view/Entry/181604?rskey= lenKD1&result=2 (accessed August 29, 2014). Also: "sleep, v."*OED Online.* http://www.oed.com/view/Entry/181603?rskey=PjsC9E&result=1 (accessed August 29, 2014).

Oxford Spanish Dictionary. 2003. New York: Oxford University Press.

Pace-Schott, Edward F. and J. Allan Hobson. 2002. "The Neurobiology of Sleep: Genetics, Cellular Physiology and Subcortical Networks." *Nature Reviews/ Neuroscience* 3 (August): 591–605.

Shakespeare, William. 2012. *The Tragedy of Hamlet, Prince of Denmark.* Folger Shakespeare Library, edited by Barbara A. Mowat and Paul Werstine. New York: Simon & Schuster.

Sinton, C. M and McCarley, R. W. 2004. "Neurophysiological Mechanisms of Sleep and Wakefulness: A Question of Balance." *Seminars in Neurology* 24 (3) (Sept): 211–213.

Sterpenich, Virginie, Genevieve Albouy, Annabelle Darsaud, Christina Schmidt, Gilles Vandewalle, Thien Thanh Dang Vu, Martin Desseilles, Christophe Phillips, Christian Degueldre, Evelyne Balteau, Fabienne Collette, Andre Luxen, and Pierre Maquet. 2009. "Sleep Promotes the Neural Reorganization of Remote Emotional Memory." *The Journal of Neuroscience* 29 (16) (April 22): 5143–5152.

Takahara, Madoka, Hiroshi Nittono, and Tadao Hori. 2002. "Comparison of the Event-Related Potentials Between Tonic and Phasic Periods of Rapid Eye Movement Sleep." *Psychiatry and Clinical Neurosciences* 56: 257–258.

The Holy Bible, King James Version. 1988. Nashville: Holman.

The New England Primer. 1784. Philadelphia, PA: B. Franklin and D. Hall.

Tononi, Giulio and Chiara Cirelli. 2003. "Sleep and Synaptic Homeostasis: A Hypothesis." *Brain Research Bulletin* 62: 143–150.

Ward, Andrew M., Donald G. McLaren, Aaron P. Schultz, Jasmeer Chhawal, Brendon P. Boot, Trey Hedden, and Reisa A. Sperling. 2013. "Daytime Sleepiness is Associated with Decreased Default Mode Network Connectivity in Both Young and Cognitively Intact Elderly Subjects." *Sleep* 36 (11): 1609–1615B.

Wehrle, Renate, Christian Kaufmann, Thomas C. Wetter, Florian Holsboer, Dorothee P. Auer, Thomas Pollmacher, and Michael Czisch. 2007. "Functional Microstates Within Human REM Sleep: First Evidence from fMRI of a Thalamocortical Network Specific for Phasic REM Periods." *European Journal of Neuroscience* 25: 863–871.

Werth, Esther, Peter Achermann, and Alexander A. Borbely.1997. "Fronto-Occipital EEG Power Gradients in Human Sleep." *Journal of Sleep Research* 6: 102–112.

Xie, Lulu, Hongyi Kang, Qiwu Xu, Michael J. Chen, Yonghong Liao, Meenakshisundaram Thiyagarajan, John O'Donnell, Daniel J. Christensen, Charles Nicholson, Jeffrey J. Iliff, Takahiro Takano, Rashid Deane, and Maiken Nedegaard. 2013. "Sleep Drives Metabolite Clearance from the Adult Brain." *Science* 342 (October 18): 373–376.

Yang, Guang, Cora Sau Wan Lai, Joseph Cichon, Lei Ma, Wei Li, and Wen-Biao Gan. 2014. "Sleep Promotes Branch-Specific Formation of Dendritic Spines after Learning." *Science* 344 (6188): 1173–1178.

3   What is Hypnosis?

What is hypnosis? One answer: "Seventy years of amazement, and still don't know what it is!" That was the title of a speech by John G. (Jack) Watkins, Ph.D., one of the great pioneers in the study and practice of hypnosis in the United States.[1]

As the recipient of the 2009 Dr. Bernauer W. Newton Award, he was asked to address the annual convention of the American Society of Clinical Hypnosis (ASCH) in Boston. At the time, Dr. Watkins was Professor Emeritus of Clinical Psychology, University of Montana, and provided a mesmerizing overview of seven decades in the use of hypnosis in America. To define or even to describe this complex yet enormously useful field has been a challenge to all who have chosen to work with it.

The use of various forms of hypnotic techniques can be traced back thousands of years. Hypnosis – often known by different names – has been practiced in one form or another in conjunction with the earliest forms of worship, of attempts at healing mental and physical ills, and through all kinds of efforts to communicate with or understand the mysteries of what was believed to exist beyond life on earth. Were these activities really what we consider to be "hypnosis"? Hypnosis has been misrepresented, misunderstood, and maligned. False, preposterous claims have been made and strange results have been attributed to hypnosis. Beyond its use and exploitation as a form of entertainment (often through scenes of ridicule or humiliation), hypnosis has also been associated with a perception of dark and nefarious uses. Quite frequently these many different perceptions have overshadowed the real answer to the question: *What is hypnosis?*

A good starting point is an answer offered in 1943 by Dr. G.H. Estabrooks, then Professor of Psychology at Colgate University:

> Genuine hypnotism actually stands in the same category as chemistry, physics or mathematics. It is based on definite basic laws and principles which have been discovered by patient experiment and research; and just as astronomy has evolved from the superstitions of astrology, and chemistry from the medieval search for the magical "philosopher's stone," so hypnotism has evolved from

the "mesmerism" of the eighteenth and nineteenth centuries into a true science, a branch of the great subject of the human brain and human consciousness.

(Estabrooks 1957, 1)

What is Hypnosis? Attempts to Describe and Define

Hypnosis cannot be seen, heard, or touched. Until very recently it could only be described or felt, often only through the eyes of an observer or through speculation about certain results that were sometimes, but not always, visible. Such descriptions and documentation of hypnosis were limited: whether oral or written, until very recently all were mere attempts at describing hypnosis or its effects, real or imagined. There were no photographs, film, or electronic recorded images of any kind that could document the physiological changes occurring during the process of hypnosis. With the invention of sophisticated instruments to record and measure such physiological changes occurring in the brain, it is now possible to begin to understand the underlying biological substrate of hypnosis. *Being in a "hypnotic state" is a clearly identifiable state which can now be measured and recorded through scientific instruments.*

These new tools and other technological advances have recently allowed us to be able to look inside the brain and see what changes are occurring in neuronal function. We can actually see and document the physiological changes that occur during hypnosis and which are specific to the hypnotic state. This chapter will show images obtained through technologically advanced techniques – including functional magnetic resonance imaging (fMRI), positron emission tomography (PET) and spectral electroencephalogram (EEG) analysis – which illustrate the actual physiological changes that occur in the brain when entering the state of hypnosis as well as during hypnosis. This is why we might wish to consider the age in which we currently live as witnessing the beginning of a new science of hypnosis.

Additionally, similar leaps – for similar reasons – are occurring in our understanding of the brain. These parallel, concurrent, and interconnected advances concurrently result in breakthroughs which lead to unexpected discoveries. For instance, in *The Induction of Hypnosis* (1986), William E. Edmonston, Jr. (who became Erickson's successor in 1968 as Editor of the *American Journal of Clinical Hypnosis* (AJCH)) wrote that "interest in the eyes as indicators both of the presence of hypnosis and the capacity for hypnosis continues." He added that:

> From the earlier chapters of this book, we are familiar with the central focus held by the eyes in the induction of hypnosis. Hull, 1933, . . . measured the capacity for hypnosis by calculating how long it took the eyelids to close during eye-fixation, eye-closure suggestions.
>
> (Edmonston 1986)

Finally, summarizing:

> The main thrust of all these studies has been to assess cerebral hemispheric activity through eye movements. The eyes, the only naturally visible part of the central nervous system, continued to hold our attention, as they did for the ancients. It may well be that through the eyes will come our understanding of hypnosis and hypnotizability.

This book is about hypnosis and its use in sleep medicine. The words hypnosis and sleep are entwined both mythologically and scientifically with myths dating back millennia. As mentioned in Chapter 2, among the most delightful and popular stories from Greek mythology is that of Hypnos, the god of sleep, known in Rome as Somnus or Sopor.

In the nineteenth century, James Braid coined the term "hypnosis," a term which continues to be used up to the present time (Olness and Kohen 1996, 11–13). He was impressed with the tendency of the hypnotized subject to sleep and regarded hypnosis as a form of sleep. Hypnosis is now recognized as a distinctly different condition than sleep. However, it is interesting to note that hypnotized patients may drift into a deep hypnotic sleep spontaneously.

Despite the rapidly increasing number of research projects and sophisticated experiments around the globe, there continues to be a lack of agreement as to *what hypnosis is*. Definitions abound and complaints about the inadequacy of these definitions continue. A great number of competing theoretical models and explanations flourish.

D. Corydon Hammond offers a very encouraging and positive response to these diverse and, at times, seemingly contradictory definitions. He believes that these "competing theories should be viewed as complementary perspectives rather than as exclusive or competing dimensions." He explains further through the following summary:

> Personally, I believe hypnotic response is a multidimensional equation that varies from person to person. It likely consists of physiological and state variables (e.g. dissociative capacity, genetically endowed aptitude, capacity to flexibly control brainwave states), cognitive variables (e.g. imaginative strategies, absorption, fading of reality orientation), and contextual–interpersonal variables (e.g.. relationship factors, reinforcement, transference, cultural role conceptions, history of abuse).

> (Hammond 1998, 1)

Current Definitions of Hypnosis

Among the many and various definitions of hypnosis the following are the most widely accepted.

In 2014, the American Psychological Association's Society of Psychological Hypnosis (APA Division 30; www.facebook.com/APA Div30/) offered the following definitions on its website (psychological hypnosis.com):

> **Hypnosis:** A state of consciousness involving focused attention and reduced peripheral awareness characterized by an enhanced capacity for response to suggestion.
> **Hypnotic induction**: A procedure designed to induce hypnosis.
> **Hypnotizability:** An individual's ability to experience suggested alterations in physiology, sensations, emotions, thoughts, or behavior during hypnosis.
> **Hypnotherapy:** The use of hypnosis in the treatment of a medical or psychological disorder or concern.

On its website (asch.net) the ASCH states that "Hypnosis is a state of inner absorption, concentration and focused attention" and further defines it through a discussion of how it is used today through a summary of the views generally accepted by its membership. According to ASCH, "recent research supports the view that hypnotic communication and suggestions effectively changes aspects of the person's physiological and neurological functions."

The Society for Clinical and Experimental Hypnosis defines hypnosis on its website (sceh.us) as a:

> state of focused attention and receptivity which can be an extremely useful tool for individuals wishing to master certain abilities and accomplish specific tasks. It has a long history, going back hundreds of years, it was originally used by clergymen, physicians, neurologists, psychologists, and others involved in the healing arts. Currently it is most competently used by healthcare professionals and mental health specialists in assisting with a broad variety of problems and life issues.

And:

> Hypnosis is considered to be a normal and adaptive altered state of consciousness that occurs spontaneously for many individuals throughout life.
>
> (sceh.us)

A very useful source for definitions and descriptions of modern hypnosis are the The Willmarth Hypnosis Interviews, many of which can be found on www.hypnosiscentral.com. They are selected from more than 100 interviews by the psychologist Eric K. Willmarth, Ph.D. Over the years Dr. Willmarth has interviewed some of "the greatest living hypnosis researchers and clinicians" and these short video interviews have been preserved in his collection.[2]

In the simplest terms, hypnosis can be summarized as an altered state of awareness that has the following three essential components: (1) suggestibility; (2) dissociation; and (3) focused attention.

Among the respected authors and practitioners of hypnosis who have offered their own – at times unique – views of hypnosis are the following.

Milton Erickson, one of the American pioneers of hypnotherapy and the founder and first president of the ASCH wrote that the:

> hypnotic state is an experience that belongs to the subject, derives from the subject's own accumulated learning and memories, not necessarily consciously recognized but possible of manifestation in a special state of non-waking awareness. Hence the hypnotic trance belongs only to the subject, the operator can do no more than learn how to proffer stimuli and suggestions to evoke responsive behavior based upon the subject's own experiential past.
>
> (Erickson and Rossi 1977, 40)

Bernauer "Fig" Newton, founder of the Newton Center for Clinical Hypnosis in Los Angeles, related that "hypnotherapy is not a single thing, is applicable to all orientations and specialties, and facilitates the efforts of a good therapist – not a substitute" (personal notes to Dr. Kohler from Dr. Newton).

The hypnotherapist Herbert Spiegel defined hypnosis as:

> a psychophysiological set characterized by a complex perceptual capacity for attentive, receptive concentration with parallel awareness. That is, the subject can be aware of a perceptual set and, at the same time, feel along side the set. Perhaps to highlight this feature, a more accurate label for the hypnotic phenomenon would be "paragnosis."
>
> (Spiegel 1981, 339)

Martin Orne, past editor of *The International Journal of Clinical and Experimental Hypnosis,* has stated that: "In its simplest form one would define hypnosis as that state or condition which exists when appropriate suggestions will elicit hypnotic phenomena. Hypnotic phenomena are then defined as positive responses to test suggestions" (Orne 1977, 18).

Marc Oster, past president of ASCH, defined hypnosis as:

> the outcome of a collaborative interpersonal relationship in which one individual, the therapist, facilitates in the other person, a patient or client, an experience that enables the client or patient to be open to changes in their thought, feelings or behaviors. This process

usually involves three elements in the subject: an ability to focus their attention or to concentrate, the ability to separate themselves from surrounding distractions, and an increase in their receptiveness to suggestion.

(marcoster.homestead.com)

There are numerous physiological and behavioral theories seeking to explain hypnosis. Many respected works provide excellent descriptions of these many, at times, conflicting theories. Most of the work in the field of hypnotherapy (hypnosis in medicine) has been done since 1953. Behavioral theories include: sleep state theory, hypnosis as a modified or special state of consciousness, hypnosis as an atavistic phenomenon, psychoanalytically oriented theories, hypnosis as a dissociative condition, and ego state theory. In "Medical Hypnosis: An Introduction and Clinical Guide," Roberta Temes, Ph.D., provides an overview and has assembled an excellent collection of essays.[3]

Hypnosis is a safe, effective technique when utilized by a trained professional within the practitioner's scope of practice. As any other medical technique, it should only be used by those who have the necessary clinical skills. A summary of possible complications and dangers of hypnosis is reported by Frank MacHovec (1988) in the AJCH. A more recent compilation of articles in a special issue of the AJCH (July 2012) focuses on a discussion of the most common concerns in the areas of clinical and forensic hypnosis. It includes six essays on the topic of "Minimizing the Risk of Inadvertent Consequences of Hypnosis: Clinical and Forensic Applications."

As predicted more than half a century ago by Estabrooks, hypnosis has the potential for significantly improving our lives (Estabrooks 1957). With the scientific advancements in our understanding of the underlying neural substrate for hypnosis and the appropriate application to clinical practice, hypnosis will play an even greater role in the physician's armamentarium.

What is Hypnosis? The Physiology of Hypnosis

In this segment we will look at the underlying neural mechanisms of hypnosis.

With the advent of more sophisticated analytical and diagnostic tools brain function can be analyzed more precisely and can begin to show the unique changes in the brain that occur during hypnosis. Historically, the use of hypnosis has been held back and diminished because of its lack of acceptance by mainstream clinicians and researchers. More recent neural imaging techniques have opened opportunities to utilize hypnosis as a research tool looking into brain mechanisms as well as the underlying substrate of hypnosis itself. Utilizing EEG, PET, and fMRI, specific physiological

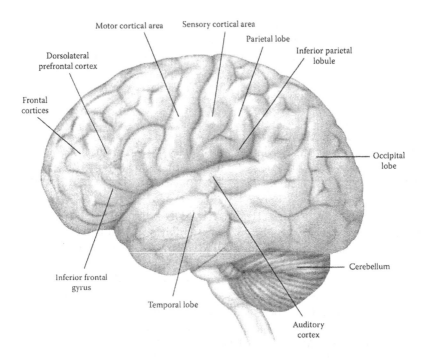

Figure 3.1 Lateral view of brain with key parts which will be mentioned in subsequent paragraphs.

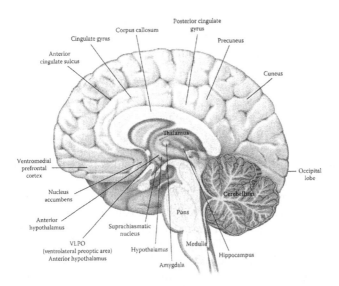

Figure 3.2 Sagittal cut of brain with key parts which will be mentioned in subsequent paragraphs.

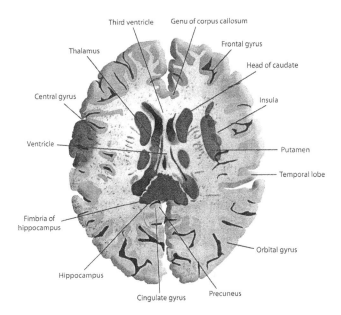

Figure 3.3 Horizontal cut of brain with key parts which will be mentioned in subsequent paragraphs.

changes in the brain associated with hypnosis can now be documented. The various EEG and imaging studies are technically very difficult because verbal and non-verbal cues can affect brain activity. This may produce results that are not a direct reflection of experimental suggestion.

Rainville et al. utilized PET measuring regional cerebral blood flow (rCBF) and EEG measures of brain electrical activity to study eight subjects who had moderate to high hypnotic susceptibility scores on the Stanford Hypnotic Susceptibility Scale Form A (SHSS-A). Hypnosis showed "significant increases in both occipital rCBF and delta EEG activity which were highly correlated with each other." They further found that:

> peak increases in rCBF were also observed in the caudal part of the right anterior cingulate sulcus and bilaterally in the inferior frontal gyri. Hypnosis-related decreases in rCBF were found in the right inferior parietal lobule, left precuneus, and the posterior cingulate gyrus. Hypnosis with suggestions produced additional widespread increases in rCBF in the frontal cortices predominantly on the left side.

They also found that "the medial and lateral posterior parietal cortices showed suggestion-related increases overlapping partly with regions of hypnosis-related decreases."

They suggested that their results supported:

> a state theory of hypnosis in which occipital increases in rCBF and delta activity reflect the alteration of consciousness associated with decreased arousal and possible facilitation of visual imagery. Frontal increases in rCBF associated with suggestions for altered perception might reflect the verbal mediation of the suggestions, working memory, and top-down processes involved in the reinterpretation of the perceptual experience.
>
> (Rainville et al. 1999, 110)

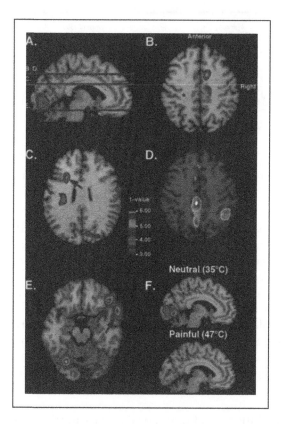

Figure 3.4 Statistical (*t*) maps of hypnosis-related increases in regional cerebral blood flow (rCBF), across stimulation conditions, in occipital (A: left 6.7), right anterior cingulate (B: superior +42.0), left frontal (arrow in C: superior +27.0), right frontal and right temporal cortices (arrows in E: superior –16.5). Decreases in blood flow were found in right lateral and medial posterior parietal cortices (D: superior +42.0; *t* color scale reversed in D). When analyzed separately in each stimulation condition, the hypnosis-related increase in occipital rCBF was observed mainly in the neutral stimulation condition, as shown in F. Coordinates refer to the atlas of Talairach and Tournoux (1988). (See Plate 3.)

Faymonville, Boly, and Laureys evaluated rCBF in healthy volunteer subjects and compared the hypnotic state with induction and suggestions for pleasant autobiographical memories to a control condition with the subject listening to autobiographical material.

> The results showed that listening to autobiographical material activates the anterior part of both temporal lobes, basal forebrain structures and some left mesiotemporal areas. During hypnosis, compared to our control task, a vast activation was observed that involved occipital, parietal, precentral, prefrontal, and cingulate cortices. The neural network implicated in hypnosis and in the control task (i.e., the evocation of autobiographical information in a state of normal alertness) did not overlap. These results show that the hypnotic state relies on cerebral processes different from simple evocation of episodic memory and suggest it is related to the activation of sensory and motor cortical areas, as during perceptions or motor acts, without actual external inputs or outputs.
>
> (Faymonville, Boly, and Laureys 2006, 464)

Raz, Fan, and Posner discussed the use of fMRI and event-related potentials in evaluating the link between attentional and hypnotic mechanisms. They also reported on a polymorphism in the COMT gene to be related to hypnotizability. They concluded: "hypnosis is a complex phenomenon likely to be associated with many genetic polymorphisms." They related: "our collective results support a potential common mechanism

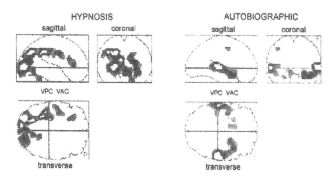

Figure 3.5 These positron emission tomography scan images show changes in regional blood flow during hypnosis compared to mental imaging of autobiographical memories. VAC, ventral anterior cingulate; VPC, ventromedial prefrontal cortex. (Reproduced from Faymonville, M., M. Boly, and S. Laureys. 2006. "Functional Neuroanatomy of the Hypnotic State." *Journal of Physiology-Paris* 99 (4–6): 463–469, with permission from Elsevier.)

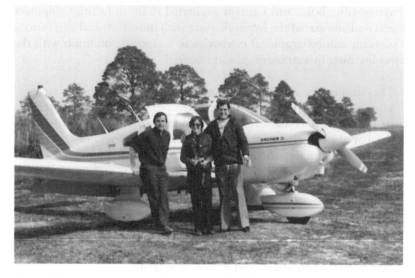

Plate 1 Family photograph taken during the 1970s. From left to right: Peter J. Kurz, Barbara B. Kohler, and her husband, Dr. William C. Kohler. By then, both Dr. and Mrs. Kohler had earned their pilot's licenses and this photograph was taken at the Kohler family airstrip in Keaton Beach, Florida (still active today as private airfield 6FL4).

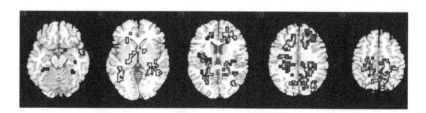

Plate 2 Brain regions which decrease activation to passive stimulation with increasing depth of hypnosis. (Reproduced from Deeley, Quinton, David A. Oakley, Brian Toone, Vincent Giampietro, Michael J. Brammer, Steven C.R. Williams, and Peter W. Halligan. 2012. "Modulating the Default Mode Network Using Hypnosis." *International Journal of Clinical and Experimental Hypnosis* 60 (2): 217, with permission of the publisher, Taylor and Francis: http://www.tandfonline.com.)

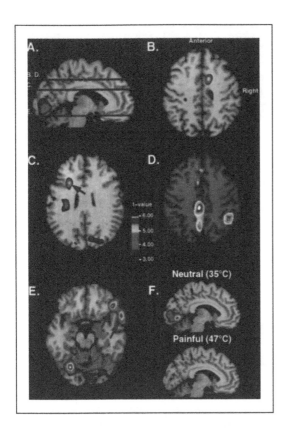

Plate 3 Statistical (*t*) maps of hypnosis-related increases in regional cerebral blood flow (rCBF), across stimulation conditions, in occipital (A: left 6.7), right anterior cingulate (B: superior +42.0), left frontal (arrow in C: superior +27.0), right frontal and right temporal cortices (arrows in E: superior −16.5). Decreases in blood flow were found in right lateral and medial posterior parietal cortices (D: superior +42.0; *t* color scale reversed in D). When analyzed separately in each stimulation condition, the hypnosis-related increase in occipital rCBF was observed mainly in the neutral stimulation condition, as shown in F. Coordinates refer to the atlas of Talairach and Tournoux (1988).

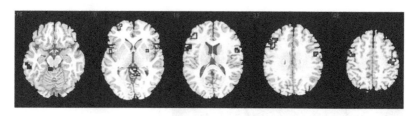

Plate 4 Brain regions which increase activation to passive visual stimulation with increasing depth of hypnosis. (Reproduced from Deeley, Quinton, David A. Oakley, Brian Toone, Vincent Giampietro, Michael J. Brammer, Steven C.R. Williams, and Peter W. Halligan. 2012. "Modulating the Default Mode Network Using Hypnosis." *International Journal of Clinical and Experimental Hypnosis* 60 (2): 217, with permission of the publisher, Taylor and Francis : http://www. tandfonline.com.)

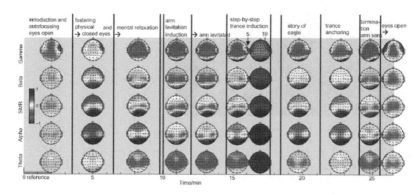

Plate 5 These spectrograms demonstrate the progression of changes which occur in the brain in each phase of hypnotic induction: prior to, during, and termination of hypnosis. The images show electroencephalogram changes utilizing power-spectoral analysis. SMR, sensorimotor rhythm. (Reproduced from Hinterberger, Thilo, Julian Schoner, and Ulrike Halsband. 2011. "Analysis of Electrophysiological State Patterns and Changes During Hypnosis Induction." *Journal of Clinical and Experimental Hypnosis* 59 (2: 170), with permission of the publisher, Taylor and Francis: http://www.tanf.co.uk/journals.)

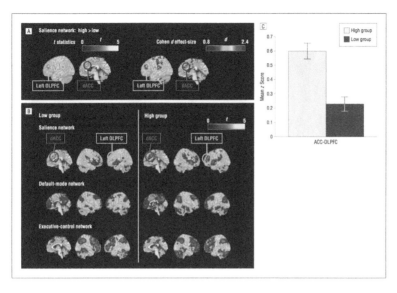

Plate 6 Significant changes in activity can be seen between the low and high hypnotizabilty groups in the dorsal lateral prefrontal cortex and the dorsal anterior cingulate cortex. Significantly higher connectivity was present in the high compared to the low hypnotizability groups. (Reproduced from Hoeft, Fumiko, John D.E. Gabrieli, Susan Whitfield-Gabrieli, Brian W. Haas, Roland Bammer, Vinod Menom, and David Spiegel. 2012. "Fuctional Brain Basis of Hypnotizability." *Archives of General Psychiatry* 69 (10) (October): 1068, with permission. Copyright © 2012 American Medical Association.)

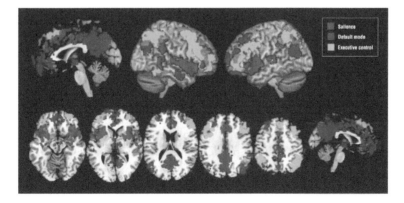

Plate 7 Functional magnetic resonance images showing the areas of the brain comprising the salience, default mode, and executive control networks. (Reproduced from Hoeft, Fumiko, John D.E. Gabrieli, Susan Whitfield-Gabrieli, Brian W. Haas, Roland Bammer, Vinod Menom, and David Spiegel. 2012. "Fuctional Brain Basis of Hypnotizability." *Archives of General Psychiatry* 69 (10) (October): 1065, with permission. Copyright © 2012 American Medical Association.)

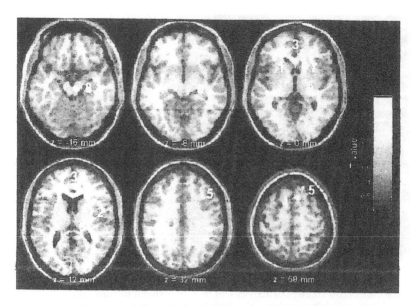

Figure 3.6 Positron emission tomographty scan images showing hypnosis-related
increased functional connectivity with midcingulate cortex: (1) left
insula; (2) right insula; (3) perigenual cortex; (4) pre-supplementary
motor cortex; (5) superior frontal gyrus; (6) right thalamus; (7) right
caudate nucleus; (8) midbrain/brainstem. (Reproduced from
Faymonville, M., M. Boly, and S. Laureys. 2006. "Functional
Neuroanatomy of the Hypnotic State." *Journal of Physiology-Paris*
99 (4–6): 463–469, with permission from Elsevier.)

of dopaminergic modulation affecting both performance on attentional
tasks and hypnotizability" (Raz, Fan and Posner 2006, 489).

Kirenskaya et al. (2011) evaluated 31 subjects utilizing EEG spectral
analysis. Based on the SHSS, 19 had high hypnotizability and 12 low hypnotizability. The analysis was carried out in the resting state without the
use of hypnosis. There were clearly marked differences between the high
and low hypnotizability subjects. In the high hypnotizability subjects, theta
range spectral power was higher and that of beta and gamma lower compared to the low hypnotizability participants. The origin of EEG rhythms
and their association with specific cognitive processes differ. Alpha and
theta activity originates from subcortical and cortical network interaction.
Alpha activity is associated with thalamocortical feedback loops and theta
activity with hippocampal–neocortical feedback loops. Alpha activity is
maximal with the subjects' eyes closed in the resting relaxed state. Theta
activity is associated with visuospatial and emotional processing, virtual
navigation, and imagery along with episodic memory processing. Beta and
gamma frequencies are generated potentially in the cortex and are felt to
play an important role during attention and higher cognitive function.

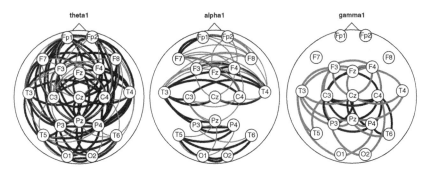

Figure 3.7 These topographic representations of the theta, alpha, and gamma
electroencephalogram frequencies show increased coherence in the theta
and alpha range for high versus low hypnotizable subjects. The authors
of this 2011 article point out that such images were not possible until
the recent availability of the "appropriate computer power to perform
coherence analysis." (Reproduced from Kirenskaya, Anna V., Vladimir
Y. Novototsky-Vlasov, and Vyacheslav M. Zvonikov. 2011. "Waking
EEG Spectral Power and Coherence Differences Between High and
Low Hypnotizable Subjects." *International Journal of Clinical and
Experimental Hypnosis* 59 (4): 442, 448, with permission from Taylor
and Francis Ltd, www.tandf.co.uk/journals.)

Hoeft et al. (2012), utilizing fMRI and structural MRI, evaluated 12 adults
with high hypnotizability and 12 with low hypnotizability. He found that
the high hypnotizability individuals had:

> greater functional connectivity between the left dorsolateral prefron-
> tal cortex, an executive control region of the brain, and the salience
> network composed of the dorsal anterior cingulate cortex, anterior
> insula, amygdala, and ventral striatum, involved in detecting, inte-
> grating, and filtering relevant somatic, autonomic, and emotional
> information using independent component analysis.
>
> (Hoeft et al. 2012, 1064)

The default mode network (DMN) was also evaluated. (The DMN
involves cortical midline structures, including medial prefrontal cortex,
superior frontal cortex, anterior cingulate cortex, posterior cingulate
cortex, precuneus, and retrosplenial cortex, along with parahippocampal gyri and lateral parietal cortices. The DMN is more active at rest
and during low demand compared to high demand or goal-directed task
conditions. It has been linked to processes such as somatic processing,
self-awareness, and task-independent thinking. It is so named because
it is active when subjects are not engaged in a particular task-oriented
activity.) Functional connectivity within the DMN did not differ reliably
between the high hypnotizability and low hypnotizability groups.

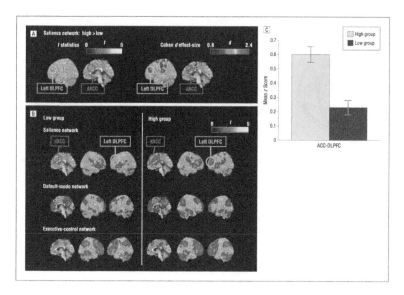

Figure 3.8 Significant changes in activity can be seen between the low and high hypnotizabilty groups in the dorsal lateral prefrontal cortex and the dorsal anterior cingulate cortex. Significantly higher connectivity was present in the high compared to the low hypnotizability groups. (Reproduced from Hoeft, Fumiko, John D.E. Gabrieli, Susan Whitfield-Gabrieli, Brian W. Haas, Roland Bammer, Vinod Menom, and David Spiegel. 2012. "Fuctional Brain Basis of Hypnotizability." *Archives of General Psychiatry* 69 (10) (October): 1068, with permission. © 2012 American Medical Association.) (See Plate 6.)

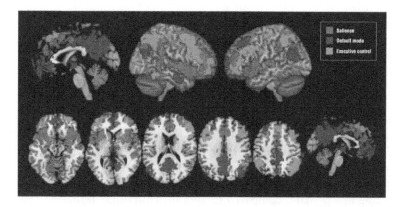

Figure 3.9 Functional magnetic resonance images showing the areas of the brain comprising the salience, default mode, and executive control networks. (Reproduced from Hoeft, Fumiko, John D.E. Gabrieli, Susan Whitfield-Gabrieli, Brian W. Haas, Roland Bammer, Vinod Menom, and David Spiegel. 2012. "Fuctional Brain Basis of Hypnotizability." *Archives of General Psychiatry* 69 (10) (October): 1065, with permission. © 2012 American Medical Association.) (See Plate 7.)

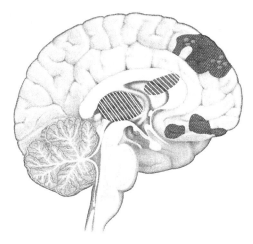

Figure 3.10 Functional magnetic resonance imaging change differences between high suggestible subjects (///) and low suggestible subjects (\\\\) in the default mode network. The most significant differences are shown in (ooo). (Reproduced from McGeown, William J., Guiliana Mazzoni, Annalena Venneri, and Irving Kirsch. 2009. "Hypnotic Induction Decreases Anterior Default Mode Activity." *Consciousness and Cognition* 18: 853, with permission.)

McGeown et al., utilizing fMRI, evaluated whether hypnosis produced a unique hypnotic state with specific neural correlates. Eleven subjects with high suggestibility and seven with low suggestibility were evaluated while engaging in visual tasks during hypnosis and also in a non-hypnotic state. Hypnosis showed a decrease in brain activity in the anterior part of the default mode circuit in the highly suggestible subjects. There were no detectable changes in this area in subjects with low suggestibility. The researchers concluded that "hypnotic induction creates a distinctive and unique pattern of brain activation in highly suggestible subjects" (McGeown et al. 2009, 848).

Deeley et al. (2012) utilized hypnosis experimentally to evaluate functioning of the DMN. Eight subjects who scored median to high hypnotizability on the Harvard Group Scale of Hypnotic Susceptibility, Form A, were evaluated utilizing fMRI pre-hypnosis, during hypnosis, and after reversal of hypnosis. The researchers relied on self-reports of hypnotic depth. Subjective hypnotic depth in the hypnosis condition differed significantly from both the pre-hypnosis condition and the post-hypnosis condition. Brain regions which demonstrated decreased activation during the passive visual stimulation with increasing depth of hypnosis included DMN regions, including cortical midline structures of the left medial frontal gyrus, right anterior cingulate gyrus, and bilateral posterior cingulate gyri along with the bilateral parahippocampal gyri.

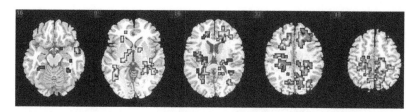

Figure 3.11 Brain regions which decrease activation to passive stimulation with increasing depth of hypnosis. (Reproduced from Deeley, Quinton, David A. Oakley, Brian Toone, Vincent Giampietro, Michael J. Brammer, Steven C.R. Williams, and Peter W. Halligan. 2012. "Modulating the Default Mode Network Using Hypnosis." *International Journal of Clinical and Experimental Hypnosis* 60 (2): 217, with permission of the publisher, Taylor and Francis, www.tandfonline.com.) (See Plate 2.)

Brain regions that showed increased activation during the passive visual stimulation with increasing depth of hypnosis included the right middle frontal gyrus, the inferior frontal gyrus bilaterally, and the pre-central gyrus bilaterally.

Hypnosis reduced activity in the DMN and in a non-goal-directed task. Increasing depth of hypnosis was associated with increased activity in lateral prefrontal regions involved in the maintenance of attention. Hypnosis was associated with increased attentional focus and decreased spontaneous thought. Neural activity in the DMN was inversely associated with attentional absorption and directly associated with spontaneous or stimulus-independent conceptual thought. As the subjects became more deeply hypnotized anterior cingulate activity decreased. Negative correlations were noted between hypnotic depth and activity in the anterior cingulate cortex. Hypnotic depth was negatively correlated to

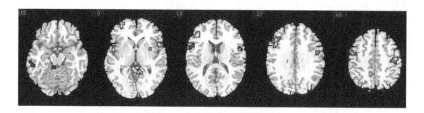

Figure 3.12 Brain regions which increase activation to passive visual stimulation with increasing depth of hypnosis. (Reproduced from Deeley, Quinton, David A. Oakley, Brian Toone, Vincent Giampietro, Michael J. Brammer, Steven C.R. Williams, and Peter W. Halligan. 2012. "Modulating the Default Mode Network Using Hypnosis." *International Journal of Clinical and Experimental Hypnosis* 60 (2): 217, with permission of the publisher, Taylor and Francis, www.tandfonline.com.) (See Plate 4.)

activity in the thalamus bilaterally. The researchers speculated that this could reflect the role of the thalamus in mediating arousal and alertness. Hypnosis was associated with reduced activity in the DMN along with increased activity in prefrontal attentional systems.

Hinterberger, Schoner, and Halsband reported on the EEG evaluation of one highly susceptible subject. Significant state changes occurred synchronously with specific induction instructions. They related: "hypnosis is not a single construct but consists of several elements such as focused attention, and awareness of internal images, the reduced ability to think critically as well as heightened compliance with suggestion" (Hinterberger, Schoner, Halsband 2011, 165). In the review they cite previous studies, at times contradictory, showing changes in the theta, beta, and gamma frequencies correlating with hypnosis. In this study, power spectral density in the bands of interest were detected utilizing a 64-channel EEG.

They found the major hypnotic state was characterized by increased frontal alpha, a decreased central, frontal, and parietal gamma in both hemispheres and an increased occipital gamma. A state of deep hypnotic trance occurred that was characterized by a strong overall heightened activity in all frequency bands.

Cojan et al. utilized topographical EEG analysis technique to investigate neural processes activated in different hypnotic and baseline conditions. Hypnotic paralysis was associated with distinctive changes in the right inferior frontal cortex. They concluded that "results add

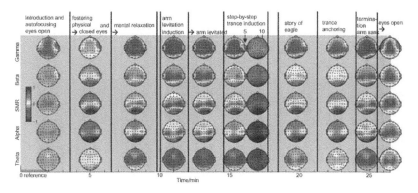

Figure 3.13 These spectrograms demonstrate the progression of changes which occur in the brain in each phase of hypnotic induction: prior to, during, and termination of hypnosis. The images show electroencephalogram changes utilizing power-spectoral analysis. SMR, sensorimotor rhythm. (Reproduced from Hinterberger, Thilo, Julian Schoner, and Ulrike Halsband. 2011. "Analysis of Electrophysiological State Patterns and Changes During Hypnosis Induction." *Journal of Clinical and Experimental Hypnosis* 59 (2: 170), with permission of the publisher, Taylor and Francis, www.tanf.co.uk/journals.) (See Plate 5.)

support to the view that hypnosis might act by enhancing executive control systems mediated by right prefrontal areas, but does not produce paralysis via direct motor inhibition processes normally used for the voluntary suppression of actions" (Cojan et al. 2013, 423).

Cardena et al. utilized spectral analysis to evaluate EEG frequency changes in low, medium, and high hypnotizability individuals. They used EEG to record brain activity in either a normal baseline condition or during unilateral paralysis caused by hypnotic suggestion. Depth of hypnosis correlated moderately to strongly with power of the fast EEG frequencies of beta-2, beta-3, and gamma. They concluded that "hypnotic depth and spontaneous phenomena following a neutral hypnotic induction vary as a function of hypnotizability related to global functional connectivity and EEG band wave activity" (Cardena et al. 2013, 375).

Muller et al. conducted an fMRI study on 16 healthy volunteers where they were asked either to imagine or to execute repetitive finger movements during a hypnotic trance. The researchers observed:

> fMRI-signal increases exclusively related to hypnosis in the left superior frontal cortex, the left anterior cingulate gyrus and left thalamus. While the superior frontal cortex and the anterior cingulate were active related more to movement performance than to imagery, the thalamus was activated only during motor imagery. These areas represent central nodes of the salience network linking primary and higher motor areas.

They concluded that "our data substantiate the notion that hypnosis enhances motor imagery" (Muller et al. 2012, 164).

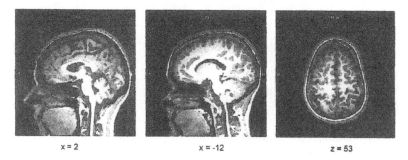

x = 2   x = -12   z = 53

Figure 3.14 Enhanced activity in the right anterior caudate gyrus, the left superior frontal gyrus, and the left thalamus during hypnosis compared to control conditions. (Reproduced from Muller, Katharina, Katrin Bacht, Stephanie Schramm, and Rudiger J. Seitz. "The Facilitating Effect of Clinical Hypnosis on Motor Imagery: An fMRI Study." *Behavioral Brain Research* 231: 666, with permission from Elsevier.)

In 2011 Raz reviewed the pertinent research up to that time on neural imaging techniques and concluded that, "while recent brain imaging research increasingly incorporates variations of suggestion and hypnosis, correlating overarching hypnotic experiences with specific brain substrates remained tenuous." Significant research findings have been made since that time period. Support for a distinctive physiological marker of trance or altered state of consciousness unique to hypnosis or to hypnotic suggestion is mounting but still not incontrovertible (Raz 2011, 363).

Hypnosis is a useful clinical tool to be utilized for clinical benefit. The development of newer diagnostic techniques along with the renewed interest in utilizing hypnosis to understand basic brain mechanisms will further advance knowledge of this fascinating clinical tool called hypnosis.

It is extremely important to continue on the current path of rapid expansion in the use of medical hypnosis. The increased use and sophistication of research studies will lead to better definitions, a more accurate description, and perhaps greater theoretical agreement. Two new factors make the current era unique.

First, even if the "why" or "how" of hypnosis is not fully comprehended, there is knowledge that hypnosis and hypnotic techniques are effective and medically beneficial to a great number of patients.

Second, in this field there is now a rapidly growing body of new research generating new evidence and a better understanding of the fact that hypnosis is a scientifically validated form of medical treatment.

Hypnosis is a uniquely altered state of consciousness with its own distinctive neural correlates. The renewed interest worldwide in using hypnosis for many and varied purposes – including medical – comes from an increasing recognition that hypnosis is not an illusion, it is not "magic" or deception, but a very real state of being which can be of great help to everyone. Because of the new, sophisticated tools and instruments which allow today's scientists to study and to document what is happening in the human brain, why it is happening, and what all this means, the related fields that study sleep and dreams also help validate and define hypnosis. What until recently could only be "described" or "felt" can now be "photographed" and documented. Increasingly, this also helps us to understand hypnosis and to develop better and better techniques to allow us to benefit from this fascinating tool called hypnosis.

In the chapters that follow, we will provide examples of the use of hypnosis in the practice of sleep medicine.

Notes

1 "Hypnosis: Seventy years of amazement, and still don't know what it is !" was an address by Jack Watkins at the 2009 convention of the American Society of Clinical Hypnosis delivered in Boston when he was awarded the 2009 Dr. Bernauer W. Newton Award. Its text was reproduced in the *American Journal of Clinical Hypnosis* (52:2, October 2009), which also included the following abstract:

This paper has reviewed the author's experience with hypnosis and related therapies from 1934 through World War II, psychological warfare, multiple personality, the origins and feuding of hypnosis societies, the development of hypnotic ego state therapy and the unique contributions of his colleague and wife, Helen Watkins.

Bernauer W. ("Fig") Newton, Ph.D. (1917–2001) was a highly respected and well-known authority in the field of hypnosis and the use of hypnotic techniques. At St. Lawrence University he earned a Bachelor of Science degree in biology, psychology, and physics (1939) and also his Master of Education degree (1940). In 1951, he received his Ph.D. in psychology at the University of California, Los Angeles. He served as president of the California Society of Clinical Hypnosis from 1977 to 1979 and as president of the Society for Clinical and Experimental Hypnosis (SCEH) from1983 to 1985.

The following biographical notes are from a eulogy (http://www.durbin hypnosis.com/obituary.htm#bernard_w._newton):

In 1959, he was one of the very early Diplomats of the American Board of Psychological Hypnosis (ABPH). His papers and chapters were numerous, reflecting his early interest in Multiple Personality Disorder (now termed Dissociative Identity Disorder), forensic hypnosis, and the "Hypnotherapist and the Cancer Patient", his 1984 SCEH presidential address. In 1983, he received the Morton Prince Award given by SCEH and awarded "for distinguished contributions to the development of hypnosis in the science and profession of psychology," and in the same year he received the Milton H. Erickson Award given by ASCH, "for excellence in scientific writing." He retired in 1989 and moved with his family to Bozeman, Montana . . . . He was a Fellow of the American Psychological Association (APA), Division 30, the American Society of Clinical Hypnosis (ASCH), and SCEH.

2 In his own words (from Dr. Willmarth's website www.hypnosiscentral.com):

I have always been fascinated by the history of hypnosis. From Franz Anton Mesmer to William James to Sigmund Freud and on to Milton Erickson, the story of hypnosis has included many of the great names in medicine, psychology, literature and politics. What other topic can bring together names such as Benjamin Franklin, Edgar Allen Poe, Wolfgang Amadeus Mozart, Charles Dickens, Marie Antoinette, Jean Marie Charcot, Ernest Hilgard and Clark Hull?

Clinical hypnosis has been attacked by the church and endorsed by a Pope. It has been acknowledged by the American Medical Association, the American Psychological Association, and the National Institutes of Health. It has been used as the sole anesthetic in thousands of medical procedures and operations, has helped to solve crimes and is used in psychotherapy to treat anxiety, depression and many other conditions. Still, there are detractors and the exact definition of hypnosis remains elusive.

3 Roberta Temes,'s collection of essays, *Medical Hypnosis: An Introduction and Clinical Guide,* is one in the series of Medical Guides to Complementary and Alternative Medicine edited by Marc S. Micozzi. Chapter 2 in the Temes volume, by Gerard Sunnen, addresses the question of "What is Hypnosis?" and provides a clear and informative overview of the topic. The chapter is followed by a comprehensive, well-selected listing of more than 100 references.

References

Braid, James. 1843. *Neurypnology, or the Rationale of Nervous Sleep.* London: J. Churchill.

Cardena, Etzel, Peter Jonsson, Devin B. Terhune, and David Marcusson-Clavertz. 2013. "The Neurophenomenology of Neutral Hypnosis." *Cortex* 49: 375–385.

Cojan, Yann, Aurelie Archimi, Nicole Chesaux, Lakshmi Waber, and Partik Vuilleumier. 2013. "Time Course of Motor Inhibition During Hypnotic Paralysis: EEG Topographical and Source Analysis." *Cortex* 49: 423–436.

Deeley, Quinton, David A. Oakley, Brian Toone, Vincent Giampietro, Michael J. Brammer, Steven C. R. Williams, and Peter W. Halligan. 2012. "Modulating the Default Mode Network Using Hypnosis." *International Journal of Clinical and Experimental Hypnosis* 60 (2): 217.

Edmonston, William E. Jr. 1986. *The Induction of Hypnosis.* New York: Wiley.

Erickson, Milton H. and Ernest L. Rossi. 1977. "Autohypnotic Experiences of Milton H. Erickson." *American Journal of Clinical Hypnosis* 20 (1): 36–54.

Estabrooks, G. H. 1957. *Hypnotism.* New York: E. P. Dutton.

Faymonville, M., M. Boly, and S. Laureys. 2006. "Functional Neuroanatomy of the Hypnotic State." *Journal of Physiology-Paris* 99 (4–6): 463–469.

Hammond, D. Corydon, ed. 1998. *Hypnotic Induction and Suggestion.* Des Plaines, Il: American Society of Clinical Hypnosis.

Hinterberger, Thilo, Julian Schoner, and Ulrike Halsband. 2011. "Analysis of Electrophysiological State Patterns and Changes During Hypnosis Induction." *Journal of Clinical and Experimental Hypnosis* 59 (2): 170.

Hoeft, Fumiko, John D. E. Gabrieli, Susan Whitfield-Gabrieli, Brian W. Haas, Roland Bammer, Vinod Menom, and David Spiegel. 2012. "Fuctional Brain Basis of Hypnotizability." *Archives of General Psychiatry* 69 (10) (October): 1068.

Kirenskaya, Anna V., Vladimir Y. Novototsky-Vlasov, and Vyacheslav M. Zvonikov. 2011. "Waking EEG Spectral Power and Coherence Differences Between High and Low Hypnotizable Subjects." *International Journal of Clinical and Experimental Hypnosis* 59 (4): 442–448.

MacHovec, Frank. 1988. "Hypnosis Complications, Risk Factors and Prevention." *American Journal of Clinical Hypnosis* 31: 40–49.

McGeown, William J., Guiliana Mazzoni, Annalena Venneri, and Irving Kirsch. 2009. "Hypnotic Induction Decreases Anterior Default Mode Activity." *Consciousness and Cognition* 18: 853.

Muller, Katharina, Katrin Bacht, Stephanie Schramm, Rudiger J. Seitz. "The Facilitating Effect of Clinical Hypnosis on Motor Imagery: An fMRI Study." *Behavioral Brain Research* 231: 666

Olness, Karen and Daniel P. Kohen. 1996. *Hypnosis and Hypnotherapy with Children,* 3rd ed. New York: Guilford Press.

Orne, Martin T. 1977. "The Construct of Hypnosis: Implications of the Definition for Research and Practice." *Annals of the New York Academy of Sciences* 296: 14–33.

Rainville, P., R. K. Hofbauer, T. Paus, G. H. Duncan, M. C. Bushnell, and D. D. Price. 1999. "Cerebral Mechanisms of Hypnotic Induction and Suggestion." *Journal of Cognitive Neuroscience* 11: 110–125.

Raz, Amir. 2011. "Does Neuroimaging of Suggestion Elucidate Hypnotic Trance?" *International Journal of Clinical and Experimental Hypnosis* 59 (3): 363–377.

Raz, Amir, Jin Fan, and Michael. I. Posner. 2006. "Neuroimaging and Genetic Associations of Attentional and Hypnotic Processes." *Journal of Physiology Paris* 99: 483–491.

Spiegel, Herbert. 1981. "Hypnosis: Myth and Reality." *Psychiatric Annals* 11 (9): 336–342.

Talairach, Jean and Pierre Tournoux. 1988. *Co-Planar Stereotaxic Atlas of the Human Brain: 3-D Proportional System: An Approach to Cerebral Imaging.* New York: Thieme Medica.

Temes, Roberta. 1998. *Medical Hypnosis: An Introduction and Clinical Guide.* New York: Churchill Livingstone.

4 A Brief History of Medical Hypnosis

The history of what we today call "hypnosis" is shaped by our understanding and definition of the meaning of "hypnotism" and "hypnotic techniques." Such definitions, the kinds of practices to which they were attached, the labels used, and their meaning at different times and in different places all create and direct the historic thread.

It is common to read about the long history of "hypnosis" with its beginning thousands of years ago, practiced by the Celts, Druids, "primitive tribes," and representatives of "ancient cultures" everywhere. We can read about the "sleep temples" of Egypt, Hindu yoga meditation, and the many ancient rituals and spiritual practices which, it is suggested, somehow appear to be related to "hypnosis." Of course, it is always added, these ancestors called the use of hypnotic practices by different names.

Yes, "more than 4,000 years ago, Wang Tai, the founder of Chinese medicine, taught a therapeutic technique that utilized incantations and manual passes over the body of the patient" (Gravitz 1991, 19). And we know that "utilizing the medium of induced states of altered awareness (trances) was practiced by the ancient Chinese, Egyptians, Hebrews, Indians, Persians, Greeks, Romans, and others" (Gravitz 1991, 19). But have these early practices and experiments truly affected our current understanding or the usefulness of "hypnosis" in the twenty-first century? It is well documented in many ways that "sleep temples" did exist in ancient Egypt, followed by one form or another of "dream healing" in Greco-Roman temples. Healing temples to the god Asclepius could be found everywhere around the Mediterranean. The nature of what was believed and practiced varied greatly depending on numerous factors, including their location. From the fifth century BC, for almost 800 years, different practices evolved in different locations. Some were strictly based on miraculous divine intervention while others also practiced surgical procedures. Frequently the inducement of sleep or trances has been misrepresented as "hypnosis" even as the purposes were misguided and in many ways the practices were misused.

Gravitz pointed out that "historians who attempt to link Asclepian healing to hypnosis usually ignore the complex and diverse nature of the

Asclepian cult and the social and cultural matrix in which it evolved" (Gravitz 1991, 46). Instead, according to Gravitz, they focus on "dream healing" which required that the patients sleep in the temple. After such sleep-overs, the expected outcome was cure by the temple god or, if the cure did not take place, a prescription provided to the supplicant for the cure (allegedly from the god).

Hypnotic State or Role Enactment?

More importantly, some of the major questions today continue to relate to the ongoing discussion among those practitioners who believe that "hypnosis is a special state of consciousness" and various behavioral theories which seek to define hypnosis as a form of "role play," determined to a great extent by consciously or, perhaps, unconsciously determined simulation. Advocates of hypnosis as a "modified" or "special" state of consciousness include James and many today, especially in the field of medicine – including Dr. Kohler – who are beginning to see documented evidence of physiological changes in the brain. Some theorists, however, believe that "hypnosis derives from deep motivations to behave like a hypnotized person should." Gerard Sunnen in "What is Hypnosis?" (Chapter 2 of *Medical Hypnosis: An Introduction and Clinical Guide* by Roberta Temes) explains: "the definition of what constitutes hypnotic behavior can be overtly or subtly communicated by our culture or by the hypnotherapist who presents cues, verbal and nonverbal, to this effect." In these interpretations, hypnotic experiences and hypnotic behavior are "actively created by subjects" (Spanos and Chaves 1991, 68). They have been broadly identified as the "social-psychological," "sociocognitive," "cognitive-behavioral," or "nonstate" theories of hypnosis (Spanos and Chaves 1991, 66).

Professor Hobson notes that, "until 1953, physiology had very little of substance to contribute to the theory and practice of altered states of consciousness" (Hobson 2001, 19). Before describing the amazing and truly revolutionary changes in our understanding since then of how the brain works, he pays homage and recognizes Freud and James for their insights in an era of "narrow" understanding:

> In retrospect, this narrowness is surprising in view of the foreshadowing of an integrationist doctrine in the monumental work of Sigmund Freud (figure 1.11) and William James (figure 1.12) at the turn or the twentieth century. Both Freud and James were by then already thoroughly persuaded that dreams, psychotic hallucinations, and quasi-religious visions all depended, somehow, on alterations in brain function. Their work foreshadows the central thesis of this book, that altered states of consciousness are the subjective concomitants of altered states of brain physiology. How did the strong

connection between these two great thinkers separate, and why did their messages get discontinued as the twentieth century moved, at its close, inexorably toward a vindication of both of them?

(Hobson 2001, 19)

In his 1953 Introduction to the first edition of *Hypnosis in Modern Medicine*, Jerome M. Schneck, M.D., explained why he assembled his impressive and informative collection of chapters about the successful use of hypnosis in the treatment of medical disorders. Each chapter was written by a specialist in a specific medical condition or field of interest. Of the 13 contributors, eight are medical doctors and the others have earned doctorates in fields related to their writing. In his Introduction, Dr. Schneck writes that:

> Over the years, tremendous strides have been made in the development of all specialties. Investigations in hypnosis have, however, continued to be weighted heavily in psychological areas so that in the field of medicine, the applications of hypnosis in psychiatry have received attention exceeding by far the interest in hypnosis as related to other specialties.
>
> (Schneck 1963, xv)

He continues by noting that "in the past few years there has been a reactivation of interest in broader hypnosis investigation" and that "with this reactivation, focus has been centered again on medical areas aside from psychiatry." Yet, he writes, these have usually been limited to the writer's own clinical experience, adding that:

> Medical practice has become too extensive and highly specialized to permit any physician or worker in an allied area to apply his experience with hypnosis to fields beyond that in which he had been especially trained or involved through special interest in addition.
>
> (Schneck 1963, xvi)

Therefore, by assembling expert contributors with extensive and successful medical experience in the use of hypnosis Dr. Schneck hoped to provide a broader overview of the uses of hypnosis in medicine. Although his work has been described as the first textbook dealing with hypnosis and the medical specialties, Dr. Schneck recognized that not all medical specialties were included:

> Ophthalmology and otolaryngology will be noted immediately by their absence and the reason for incomplete coverage in several fields is based either on data inadequate to warrant separate chapters at this time, or hypnosis workers as yet too inexperienced or not at all available to prepare chapters that would merit inclusion.
>
> (Schneck 1963, xvii)

Of particular relevance to the authors of the present volume is the total omission of sleep medicine. Dr. Schneck's 1953 "Contents" includes the following specialties by name: internal medicine and general practice; anesthesiology and surgery; dermatology; obstetrics and gynecology; psychiatry; hypnotherapy for children; dentistry; and clinical psychology. It will be decades before sleep is recognized as a medical specialty.

The treatment of sleep disorders is not a topic and, in the entire volume, *somnambulism* is mentioned only twice in the chapter on "History of Medical Hypnosis." These references were to the Marquis de Puysegur, "who observed the sleep-walking state" of a hypnotized patient (circa 1784) and called this state of trance *somnambulisme magnétique* (somnambulism).

Even after the formal recognition of sleep as a distinct medical specialty, recent comprehensive overviews written in the twenty-first century avoid the topic of how hypnosis can and should be used in the treatment of sleep disorders. An excellent updated and expanded version of the classic 1987 J. Watkins text by Arreed Barabasz and John G. Watkins (1913–2012), published in 2005, highlights the many reasons that make the medical use of hypnosis such an important option (including treatment efficacy, cost-efficiency, and even that "hypnosis is multicultural in nature"). Its Table of Contents includes chapters that focus on the successful use of hypnosis in relieving pain, in anesthesia and surgery, for childbirth pain and trauma, in internal medicine, in the treatment of dermatological disorders, in hypnodontia and in enhancing sports performance. The treatment of sleep disorders is not mentioned in the same category or at the same level.

A comprehensive and well-documented chapter in Dr. Schneck's work shows that hypnosis in medicine covers a very wide range and has been successfully practiced – and documented – by medical doctors at least since the twentieth century. Yet, despite the linkage of sleep, dreaming, and hypnosis, which has been recognized and described over thousands of years, it was not until the 1950s that credible, scientific documentation began. This is particularly the case with modern sleep medicine.

Following the discovery of rapid eye movement (REM) sleep and tied to our better understanding of how the brain works, the authors believe that a new phase has finally begun with the practical, clinical application of principles and lessons learned about the treatment of sleep disorders through hypnosis.

Before we transition to the scientific and medical aspects of such application and use, this chapter will trace a very brief summary of how the "modern" phase of this confluence of hypnosis and the science of sleep emerged. The authors' objective with this (very) brief history is to focus attention on the relatively recent developments which have led to the successful use of hypnosis and hypnotic techniques in medicine. More specifically, the focus will be on the clinical use by highly trained and experienced medical doctors of techniques that help reach desired results in the successful treatment of *certain* sleep disorders.

Moving from Mesmer to Medical Hypnosis

If we limit ourselves to "modern" hypnosis as it is generally understood or practiced in Europe and the Western hemisphere, the most logical starting point is the first "modern" physician known to have practiced and advocated the use of hypnosis in medicine. Franz Anton Mesmer (1734–1815) received his medical degree in 1766 from the prestigious University of Vienna. The German-born physician was the originator of "mesmerism" (an expression derived from his family name) which described a form of "magnetism" that included practitioners who believed in various "fluid" and "magnetic" theories which, they claimed, could influence the health of the human body.

One definition of this force (from *Encyclopedia Britannica*) is:

> **animal magnetism,** a presumed intangible or mysterious force that is said to influence human beings. The term was used by the German physician Franz Anton Mesmer to explain the hypnotic procedure that he used in the treatment of patients. (See hypnosis.) Mesmer believed that it was an occult force or invisible fluid emanating from his body and that, more generally, the force permeated the universe, deriving especially from the stars.
>
> (*Encyclopedia Britannica* 2005)

Dr. Mesmer is important in the history of medical hypnosis for several reasons beyond his theories about *magnétisme animal* (the original name, translated into English as "animal magnetism"; the origin of the use of "animal" is sometimes ascribed to the Latin root *animus* – meaning breath, consciousness, or vital power – to indicate that this presumed force was present in all beings "with breath"). His reputation was greatly enhanced and later demolished through his close connection to the Royal Court of France's King Louis XVI; his advocacy of "animal magnetism" and "mesmerism" as a healing force extended beyond medicine and hypnosis into the worlds of politics, philosophy, and literature.[1]

The very public controversy around "animal magnetism" and "mesmerism" led to the appointment in 1784 of a Royal Commission to investigate Dr. Mesmer's claims. Among the distinguished members of this commission were Benjamin Franklin (1706–1790), Antoine-Laurent Lavoisier (1713–1794), and Joseph-Ignace Guillotin (1783–1814), a respected chemist who is also well known for his invention of the guillotine. The report of the Commission concluded that it could not find any scientifically valid evidence for Dr. Mesmer's claims and that the "described effects" were a consequence of "imagination."[2]

For many reasons a global survey is beyond the scope of this chapter. Here we limit our summary to the introduction of a few extraordinary practitioners of medical hypnosis from Europe and North America and to highlight – by necessity, rather superficially – their major contributions. Consequently this is a review of only what has been conveyed to our generation through works in the major Indo-European languages.

Our focus begins with Dr. Benjamin Rush (1745–1813), the only Founding Father of the United States to have signed both the Declaration of Independence and the Constitution of the United States. Several other medical doctors will be highlighted, ending with the Swiss psychiatrist, explorer, and hypnotist Dr. Bertrand Piccard (born 1958) whose plans for the solo circumnavigation of the Earth powered exclusively by solar power from the beginning included the use of hypnosis and hypnotic techniques.

While animal magnetism was a popular, much-debated concept in Europe during the late 18th and early 19th centuries, very little information is available about its use or discussion in the United States. According to Dr. Schneck, among the respected figures who appreciated certain positive elements in Mesmer's approach was Dr. Rush, "who is generally acknowledged to have been the best known physician of his time in the United States and is regarded as the father of American psychiatry" (Schneck 1978, 9–14).

In the Abstract he summarized his 1978 article as follows:

> An early assessment of animal magnetism in the United States was provided by Benjamin Rush in 1789 and 1812. Unlike Benjamin Franklin and his colleagues on the 1784 French commission who recognized the role of imagination, yet without its potential benefits, Rush discerned the value of both suggestion and imagination in their constructive potential and incorporated them into his medical practice while rejecting Mesmer's theories and techniques. This is of additional interest because of Rush's fame as an early American physician and his position as the father of American psychiatry.
>
> (Schneck 1978, 9)

Dr. Schneck supports his conclusions in part through the contents of a 1789 lecture to medical students at the University of Pennsylvania ("Duties of a Physician") and partly through references to Dr. Rush's major work, his *Medical Inquiries and Observations Upon The Diseases of the Mind*, published in 1812 and considered to be the first textbook of psychiatry in America. In his lecture, referring to Mesmer, Dr. Rush said:

> The facts which he has established clearly prove the influence of the imagination, and will, upon diseases. Let us avail ourselves of the handle which those faculties of the mind present to us, in the strife between life and death.
>
> (Rush 1830)

Further adding:

> Does the will beget insensibility to cold, heat, hunger, and danger?
> Does it suspend pain, and raise the body above feeling the pangs of
> Indian tortures? Let us not then be surprised that it should enable the
> system to resolve a spasm, to open an obstruction, or to discharge an
> offending humour. I have only time to hint at this subject. Perhaps
> it would lead us, if we could trace it fully to some very important
> discoveries in the cure of diseases.
>
> (Rush 1789, 256–257)[3]

In Dr. Schneck's words:

> While Franklin and Rush rejected Mesmer's theoretical notions pre-
> sented in his classic 1779 dissertation (Mesmer, 1779) Rush evidently
> was capable of appreciating the potential therapeutic benefits in the
> doctor–patient relationship at the core of animal magnetism, and the
> suggestion (will) theme inherent in it, in addition to the importance
> of imagination and its possible beneficial role in treating ill patients.[4]

Dr. Rush played an extraordinarily influential role in the early history of the
United States, as well as in academics and medicine. He lost his father when
he was six years old and was brought up in Philadelphia by his mother and
also his uncle Samuel Finley, who ran an academy in Maryland and later
became president of Princeton University. He was admitted to Princeton
as a junior and graduated in 1760 when not quite 15. After formal and
informal studies as a student and an apprentice of several distinguished
doctors, in 1754 he also attended lectures in the newly formed medical
department of what later became the University of Pennsylvania. Dr. Rush
received his M.D. degree from the University of Edinburgh, Scotland (at
the time considered one of the major medical centers of the world) where
he also persuaded John Witherspoon to move to New Jersey and become
Princeton University's sixth president.

Dr. Rush continued his studies in London and Paris. Upon his return
to the United States, at the age of 23 he was appointed to the chair of
chemistry in the College of Philadelphia's medical department, becoming the first professor of chemistry in America. During his enormously
productive career his contributions ranged from political and humanitar-
ian endeavors (including active participation in anti-slavery activities) to
academics (he founded and became president of Dickinson College in
Carlisle, Pennsylvania, and was also a charter trustee of Franklin College,
later Franklin and Marshall).

During the Revolution, Dr. Rush was Surgeon-General of the Middle
Department of the Army. Returning to Philadelphia (then the medical center of America), he resumed his practice and his teaching at the

College of Philadelphia, where it is said that he taught some 3,000 medical students and doctors.

> His greatest contributions to medical science were the reforms he instituted in the care of the mentally ill during his thirty years of service as a senior physician at the Pennsylvania Hospital. In the words of one of his biographers, Dr. Carl Binger, a psychiatrist, "he took on heroic stature," substituting kindness and compassion for cruelty, and replacing routine reliance on archaic procedures by careful clinical observation and study. The year before he died, he published *Medical Inquiries and Observations upon the Diseases of the Mind,* the first textbook on psychiatry in America, which Dr. Binger called "the crowning achievement of his professional life."
>
> (Leitch 1978)

In 1965 the American Psychiatric Association (APA) honored Dr. Rush with a bronze plaque placed at his grave site in Philadelphia, naming him "Father of American Psychiatry." To this date the APA's official seal bears Dr. Rush's portrait.

As mentioned earlier, the strongly held belief that "animal magnetism" was a distinct physical force somehow similar in importance to gravity and electricity was quite prevalent in Europe during the nineteenth century. Among the best-known proponents in England was John Elliotson, M.D. (1791–1868), who believed that this force could be used for medical purposes through its transfer from magnetized bodies or through the intervention of a "magnetizer." Opposition to his views was led by Thomas Wakley (1795–1862), the "crusading editor of the *Lancet*" (Rosen 1963, 14). Partly as a result of the *Lancet*'s opposition to "Mesmeric Humbug," the practice of animal magnetism was prohibited within the North London Hospital (1838).

> To present their cause favorably, Elliotson and his supporters in 1843 started a Journal entitled *The Zoist: A Journal of Cerebral Physiology and Mesmerism, and Their Applications to Human Welfare* . . . . The purpose of the communications published in the *Zoist* was essentially propagandistic. For the most part they comprised reports on patients treated with mesmerism, testimonials and endorsements from physicians and satisfied patients, and polemics with opponents of mesmerism.
>
> (Rosen 1963, 15)

Zoist appeared as a quarterly from April, 1843, to December, 1855. Its second volume includes reports "of the use of mesmerism for venesection, dental extraction, the establishment of setons and issues, excision of tumors, amputations, and in a case of labor." The third volume "presented three further reports on surgical operations performed on patients under mesmeric anesthesia," including four "from America, two describing the removal of tumors from the neck, the third removal of a polyp from the nose, and the fourth amputation of a breast" (Rosen 1963, 16).

This same volume of *Zoist* (March, 1845, to January, 1846) also included the remarkable reports about Dr. James Esdaile (1808–1859), a skilled Scottish surgeon who worked in India from 1845 to 1851. A hospital in the state of Bengal was made available and devoted to his mesmeric practice, which included the induction of profound trance states. The articles mention "several thousand" painless operations in which Dr. Esdaile reports the application of mesmerism for surgical anesthesia. "Of these about three hundred were major operations," according to Dr. Esdaile's articles in *Zoist* and several other publications, "including amputations, lithotomy, removal of scrotal tumors, hydrocele and cataract" (Rosen 1963, 16–17).

With the discovery of ether and chloroform, suddenly hypnoanesthesia was replaced by chemoanesthesias and this pushed mesmerism from center stage.[5] The twists and turns of the history and use of mesmerism are described in fascinating detail by Dr. Rosen in his chapter on medical hypnosis, "From Animal Magnetism to Medical Hypnosis." He offers a rich collection of examples and illustrations which explain "the historical significance of the English mesmeric movement" up to the point where it transformed itself through new insights:

> This, indeed, is the historical significance of the English mesmeric movement. It focused attention on the treatment of certain conditions, which we now call neuroses, through the agency of an effective therapy; eventually, it helped to make mesmerism respectable by providing it with another name and explanation; and finally, it provided a bridge for the transmission of this new approach to France where the next stage in the development of medical hypnosis occurred.
>
> (Rosen 1963, 19)

The Scottish ophthalmologist Dr. James Braid (1795–1860) introduced a new word around 1841 – *hypnosis* – and this name has stayed with us since then. Dr. Braid derived it from "neuro-hypnotism" or nervous sleep (perhaps "sleep of the nerves") and presented his newly developed, related interpretation in *Neurypnology, or the Rationale of Nervous Sleep*. His work, published in 1843, is generally considered to be the first book on hypnosis. It is hard to overestimate the significance of this work in the history of medical hypnosis. In essence, Dr. Baird "accepted the reality of mesmeric phenomena, but rejected the theory of animal magnetism with its idea of a magnetic fluid" (Rosen 1963, 19). He believed that the results could be attributed to *suggestion* as opposed to other "magnetic" or "occult" theories proposed by "mesmerists" and "electro-biologists."

Dr. Elliotson and Dr. Braid argued their differences and continued their feud until their death. The study, discussion, and development of hypnotism and related theories next continued in France.

In his acceptance speech upon being awarded the 2009 "Fig" Newton Award, the psychologist and psychotherapist Ernest Lawrence Rossi, Ph.D., noted the link between Dr. Braid and modern neuroscience:

> The psychological level can turn on the biological activity of gene expression and activity-dependent brain plasticity in our physical brain. This is the essence of psychosocial genomics and top-down mind–body therapy! This is how modern neuroscience has validated the essence of James Braid's (1855/1970) prescient statement about "the reciprocal actions of mind and matter upon each other" quoted above.
>
> (Rossi 2009, 281)

A detailed history of the evolution of medical hypnosis and the use of hypnotic techniques in medicine is beyond the scope of this chapter. Among the several outstanding works on this topic are the four particularly well-researched, well-written, and enjoyable-to-read works mentioned in the Notes. The focus of this chapter is on presenting a selection – mostly of physicians but also of researchers and respected clinical practitioners – who have combined their enormous body of medical knowledge and experience with a serious understanding of hypnosis. During the second half of the nineteenth century, this confluence was particularly well represented in France, where two competing groups developed and practiced conflicting approaches to the use of hypnosis in medicine. In Nancy, Ambroise-August Liébeault (1823–1904) began his rural medical practice shortly after receiving his medical degree from the University of Strasbourg in 1850. His initial interest in magnetic theories was replaced by a growing belief in hypnosis. To pursue his use of medical hypnosis – which he believed in many cases to be a better alternative to drugs and physical manipulations – he provided hypnotic treatment free of charge to his poor French peasant patients. During 1882 a previously skeptical Hippolyte Bernheim (1840–1919), already a well-known professor of neurology at the nearby University of Nancy, became convinced that Dr. Liébeault's methods were effective. In 1885, he published *Suggestive Therapeutics* describing their use of hypnosis as an approach that rejected magnetism and magnetic theories. Drs. Liébeault and Bernheim "developed what came to be known as the Nancy School, a center for hypnotic practice and instruction that emphasized the concept of suggestion and taught that hypnosis was a psychological phenomenon, not a magnetic one" (Barabasz and Watkins 2005, 14).

Around the same period one of the most celebrated physicians of this time was exploring similar issues in Paris. The French neurologist

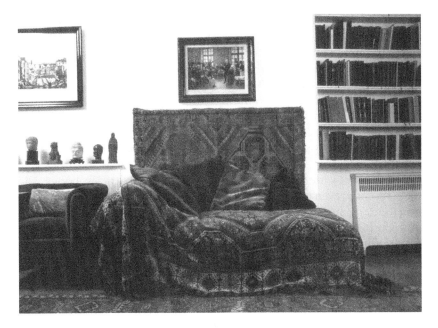

Figure 4.1 Image of Charcot's photograph above Freud's couch; from the Freud
Museum, London. Freud's study, his books, and his collection of
artifacts (assembled over his many years in Vienna) are preserved in
what is today the Freud Museum in London. Based on a careful and
comprehensive record of Freud's Vienna apartments in the weeks
before he left to resettle as a refugee in London (1938), his study is
an accurate replica which includes his original books and works of
art. The framed image above Freud's couch is a print of *Une leçon
clinique du Dr. Charcot à la Salpêtrière*, an engraving by E. Pirodon
after the oil painting by André Brouillet (1887). An excellent catalogue
with fascinating details is *Sigmund Freud and Art: His Personal
Collection of Antiquities*, edited by Lynn Gamwell and Richard Wells
and published in 1989 by Harry N. Abrams, in association with
the State University of New York and the Freud Museum, London.
(Reproduced with permission of the Freud Museum Publications.)

Jean-Martin Charcot (1825–1893) was a professor at the University of
Paris for 33 years and also had a close clinical association with the Pitié-
Salpêtrière Hospital, in Paris, ultimately becoming its Director. Among
his students, admirers, and followers were many of the leading medical
students, doctors, health workers, and intellectuals of Europe, including
William James, Pierre Janet, Sigmund Freud, and Carl Gustav Jung.

In addition to his primary focus on neurology, Dr. Charcot's research,
writings, and teaching influenced the developing fields of psychology and
psychiatry. He became known as "the founder of modern neurology."
Charcot believed that hypnotic phenomena were pathological and

"theoretically, he conceptualized hypnotism to be somatically determined, . . . a neo-mesmeric fluidist who believed that magnets, auditory stimulation, tactile pressure, and certain metals could induce a trance state" (Gravitz 1991, 21). In contrast with the group in Nancy, "he also held that hypnotism was a pathological condition of physiological and anatomical origins virtually synonymous with hysteria" (Gravitz 1991, 21). Joint experiments were set up during 1886 "to test the relative claims of each," the views of the "Nancy group prevailed, and magnetic theories of hypnotism were no longer seriously voiced after that time" (Gravitz 1991, 21). Hypnosis was established as a psychological (not magnetic) phenomenon.

Dr. Charcot's life and theories were the subject of articles, books, and more recently, even of full-length movies. Much of what has been written is inaccurate, misleading or – as in the case of a recent full-length movie – outright fiction and fabrication. *Augustine*, released in 2013 and the first feature film from the French *auteur* Alice Winocour, illustrates the difficulties faced when trying to overcome the history of misrepresentations that has created unfounded and negative connotations associated with hypnosis. Highly praised at the Cannes Film Festival as well as by many critics since then, *Augustine* benefits from an exceptionally talented cast and a superbly crafted and filmed story line. Unfortunately – and, not for the first or only time – the facts of so-called "historical documentaries" about Dr. Charcot and the Paris School are false. In a detailed review of *Augustine*, Alan A. Stone (2013) has pointed out that "Winocour knows virtually nothing about the actual relationship between Charcot and Augustine, if indeed there ever was one" and "she made the doctor–patient story up out of whole cloth." He continues, adding that "its flaws are painfully obvious and deeply troubling," "Winocour not only invented the erotic relation between Charcot and Augustine, but she also misrepresented the unfortunate young woman's history," and then decided "to fill in" voids in the hospital records "from her imagination." He summarizes by concluding that "what Winocour has done with the story of Augustine is inexcusable. If there is a moral limit to artistic license she has gone beyond it."[6]

The Beginnings of the Modern Use of Hypnosis

William James (1842–1910) never practiced medicine, yet many consider him Harvard Medical School's most distinguished graduate. In 1872 the president of Harvard invited him to teach a new course on physiology and that led to his many years of immersion as a teacher and a scholar initially in physiology and later in psychology. Upon his appointment he wrote to his brother Henry that "the appointment to teach physiology is a perfect god-send to me just now," an occupation which soon set him on course to develop a course on "The Relation Between Physiology and Psychology" and led to the establishment of the first laboratory in America for experimenting in psychology.

In 1878 James signed a contract "to produce a text-book in psychology by 1880." However, "the work grew under his hand" and was finally finished in 1890 with the publication of his two-volume *The Principles of Psychology*, (James 1890), the work that launched the field of psychology in America.

His interest in hypnosis led to Chapter XXVII, "Hypnotism," in which James described "Modes of operating and susceptibility," "Theories about the hypnotic state," and "The symptoms of the trance." He followed with interesting research on experimental psychopathology and psychotherapy and is credited with the introduction of the term "dissociation" in the field of psychiatry. In addition to his writing and teaching, Dr. James was engaged in the clinical practice of hypnosis, as confirmed in a letter to Carl Stumpf (January 1, 1886):

> I try to spend two hours a day in a laboratory for psycho-physics which I started last year, but of which I fear the fruits will be slow in ripening, as my experimental aptitude is but small. But I am convinced that one must guard in some such way as that against the growing tendency to subjectivism in one's thinking, as life goes on. I am hypnotizing, on a large scale, the students, and have hit one or two rather pretty unpublished things of which some day I hope I may send you an account . . . Ever faithfully yours, Wm. James.

In his preoccupation with better understanding "consciousness," James was curious about the implications of its relationship with hypnosis. He was familiar with the works of the pioneering French psychologist and psychotherapist Pierre Marie Félix Janet (1859–1947) and

> was persuaded by Janet's observations, and his own, that in hypnosis things could be (unconsciously) felt but not (consciously) perceived, and that mental activity could be divided into multiple streams, only one of which was accessible to phenomenal awareness at any given time.[7]

In "Hypnotism" Dr. James provides a detailed overview of the many techniques used by various practitioners of hypnosis ("each operator having his pet method") and continues with a summary of the best-known theories of the time. He lists and describes "three main opinions," the theories of:

"1 Animal magnetism" ; of
"2 Neurosis" ; and, finally, of
"3 Suggestion."

In the final section of this chapter he lists and defines "The Symptoms of the Trance," grouped as follows: amnesia; suggestibility effects on the voluntary muscles; hallucinations of all senses and delusions of every conceivable kind; real sensations may be abolished as well as false ones suggested; and hyperaesthesia of the senses. Under "Changes in the nutrition of the tissues" which "may be produced by suggestion," he lists the following – at the time quite well-known – practitioners (mostly from Europe and North America):

> These effects lead into therapeutics – a subject which I do not propose to treat of here. But I may say that there seems no reasonable ground for doubting that in certain chosen subjects the suggestion of a congestion, a burn, a blister, a raised papule, or a bleeding from the nose or skin, may produce the effect. Messrs. Beaunis, Berjon, Bernheim, Bourru, Burot, Charcot, Delboeuf, Dumontpallier, Focachon, Forel, Jendrássik, Krafft-Ebing, Liébault, Liègeois, Lipps, Mabille, and others have recently vouched for one or other of these effects.[8]

The final topics listed and described are *the post-hypnotic effects of suggestion*, and *the effects of suggestion in the waking state*. Among the additional contributions by Dr. James to the field of hypnosis is the critical listing of references and bibliographies he recommends:

> The recent literature of the subject is quite voluminous, but much of it consists in repetition. The best compendious work on the subject is *Der Hypnotismus*, by Dr. A. Moll (Berlin, 1889; and just translated into English, N.Y., 1890), which is extraordinarily complete and judicious . . . . A complete bibliography has been published by M. Dessoir (Berlin 1888).
>
> (James 1890)

Finally, Dr. James ends "Hypnosis" by noting that, "in the recent revival of interest in the history of this subject, it seems a pity that the admirably critical and scientific work of Dr. John Kearsley Mitchell of Philadelphia should remain relatively so unknown" since "it is quite worthy to rank with Braid's investigations."

Santiago Ramón y Cajal (1852–1934)

The 1906 Nobel Prize in Physiology or Medicine was awarded to the Spanish neurobiologist Santiago Ramón y Cajal (1852–1934) and Camillo Golgi, in recognition of their work "on the structure of the nervous system." However, his pioneering contributions as a neuroscientist, histologist, and pathologist had a significant and long-lasting influence in a wide range of fields. J. Allan Hobson, M.D. (born 1933),

Emeritus Professor of Psychiatry at Harvard Medical School, ranks his contributions among the "three important developments" that "set the science of sleep and dreaming on its current course." In *From Angels to Neurones*, Professor Hobson (Hobson and Wohl 2005, 130) describes the critical decade between 1890 and 1900 "in which the psychological and neurophysiological study of the brain/mind took on its current 'modern' form." Along with the publication of William James's *The Principles of Psychology* (1890) and Sigmund Freud's "completion in 1895 of the unpublished Project for a Scientific Psychology" he cites "the elaboration of the Neurone Doctrine" by Ramón y Cajal as the third key development.

Encouraged by his physician father, in 1873 Ramón y Cajal took his Licentiate in Medicine at the University of Saragossa following a successful competitive examination, and served as an army doctor. After taking part in an expedition to Cuba (1874–1875), upon his return to Spain he became an assistant in the School of Anatomy in the Faculty of Medicine at Saragossa (1875) and, at his own request, Director of the Saragossa Museum (1879). In 1877 he earned the degree of Doctor of Medicine in Madrid and was appointed Professor of Descriptive and General Anatomy at Valencia (1883), Professor of Histology and Pathological Anatomy at Barcelona (1887), and to the same Chair at Madrid (1892). He was also made honorary Doctor of Medicine of the Universities of Cambridge (1894) and Würzburg (1896) and Doctor of Philosophy of the Clark University (Worcester, United States, 1899). An avid painter, artist, and photographer he is well known for his thousands of unique and detailed histological slides and scientific drawings. Throughout his career Ramón y Cajal introduced new staining methods that enabled him to observe in detail the organization of the nervous tissue.

He is known to have studied hypnosis and there are anecdotal references to his use of hypnotic techniques in his medical and academic practice. Spanish historical records also allude to a book he wrote on the nature and potential of hypnosis. However, it is said that this work was lost or destroyed during the Spanish Civil War. According to Dr. Hobson, "a versatile and energetic man, Ramón y Cajal also practiced hypnosis" (Hobson 1988, 91).

Both Sigmund Freud (1856–1939) and Carl Gustav Jung (1875–1961) developed an interest in and, at one point or another in their celebrated lives, practiced hypnosis. Both – for different reasons – eventually abandoned the use of hypnotic techniques. Perhaps the writings of J. Allan Hobson best summarize some of the key elements of how these two giants of psychiatry and psychotherapy viewed hypnosis.

Dr. Hobson considers the Austrian neurologist and father of psychoanalysis one of the three architects of the insights and framework which, in the decade after 1890, led to "the psychological and neurophysiological study of the brain/mind" which, of course, led to "its current 'modern' form." This was particularly evident in his initially unpublished "Project for a Scientific Psychology" (1895). He writes:

> Freud, by calling attention to dreaming as a psychological model for understanding the unconscious mind in terms of its neurobiological underpinnings, foreshadowed the integrative models that can now be constructed and tested. The goals of his Project for a Scientific Psychology are finally within our grasp.
>
> (Hobson and Wohl 2005, 130)

> It is thus in a comparative spirit that I view the shared interest of Freud and Ramón y Cajal and connect it to my own perspective on hypnotic phenomena. Hypnosis is an artificially altered state of consciousness. Sleep is a naturally altered state of consciousness. Can similar rules govern the transition of state change in both the experimental and natural conditions? The fact that induction of both hypnotic and sleep states involves rhythmic stimulation and eye fixation may not be a coincidence. Both procedures may help to gain access to and control over the brain-stem centers that appear to be fundamental to conscious-state regulation.
>
> (Hobson 1988, 92)

According to Dr. Hobson, at the beginning of his career in clinical neurology Freud was "fascinated by the clinical phenomena of hypnosis and hysteria" and "dissatisfied with the model of the mind then supportable by neuroscience" (Hobson 1988, 61). In Paris, after he became familiar with Charcot's theories, he changed his career to psychiatry (then known as psychopathology). For several reasons (including his own emotional reactions to experiences with hypnotic patients), by 1896 Freud had abandoned the use of hypnosis and others quickly followed him in this rejection.

However, this did not stop the "successful application of hypnosis to numerous medical and psychological disorders" and Melvin A. Gravitz (1991) lists the following practitioners who continued its use: Morton Prince, Boris Sidis, and John Duncan Quakenbos (in the United States); Ivan Pavlov (Russia); Pierre Janet and Alfred Binet (France); C. Lloyd Tuckey, Ralph Henry Vincent, and R.W. Felkin (England); and Oskar Vogt, Rudolf Heidenhain, and Albert Moll (Germany) (Temes 1998, 30).

At the end of his life, Jung worked with Aniela Jaffe in the preparation of a wonderful volume of autobiographical essays (*Memories, Dreams, Reflections*). In this volume, the Editor and the Swiss psychiatrist and psychotherapist present valuable commentaries on some of the most important topics related to Jung's life and theories. Included is a vignette from 1905, when he became lecturer in psychiatry at the University of Zurich, as well as senior physician for four years at the Psychiatric Clinic:

During the first semesters my lectures dealt chiefly with hypnosis, also with Janet and Flournoy. Later the problem of Freudian psychoanalysis moved into the foreground. In my courses on hypnosis I used to inquire into the personal history of the patients whom I presented to the students. One case I still remember very well.

(Jung 1989, 117)

It was the case of a 58-year-old woman on crutches who had suffered for 17 years from a painful paralysis of her left leg. She told "the whole long story" of her illness until Jung said they were running out of time and "I am now going to hypnotize you." Immediately upon hearing those words she closed her eyes "and fell into a profound trance." After half an hour Jung "wanted to awaken the patient again" but "she would not wake up." Some ten minutes later "the woman came to" and "was giddy and confused."

> I said to her, "I am the doctor, and everything is all right." Whereupon she cried out, "But I am cured!" threw away her crutches, and was able to walk. Flushed with embarrassment, I said to the students, "now you've seen what can be done with hypnosis!" In fact I had not the slightest idea what had happened.
>
> That was one of the experiences that prompted me to abandon hypnosis. I could not understand what had really happened, but the woman was in fact cured, and departed in the best of spirits. I asked her to let me hear from her, since I counted on a relapse in twenty-four hours at the latest. But her pains did not recur; in spite of my skepticism, I had to accept the fact of her cure.
>
> (Jung 1989, 117)

Among the many academic environments in the United States where the study and teaching of hypnosis have flourished is Colgate University in Hamilton, New York. More than 70 years ago G.H. Estabrooks dedicated *Hypnotism*, his seminal work, to Dr. G.B. Cutten, "Former President of Colgate University and an American Pioneer in the Field of Hypnotism."

George Barton Cutten (1874–1962) was a pioneer in the use of hypnosis in the treatment of alcoholism. After earning his Ph.D. in psychology at Yale he joined the faculty of Acadia College and eventually became Acadia's president. It was at Acadia that he met and taught George H. Estabrooks (1895–1973), who enrolled at Acadia specifically to study with Cutten. After Acadia, Estabrooks spent three years as a Rhodes Scholar at Oxford and Exeter (1921–1924) and received his Ph.D. from Harvard's Graduate School of Education. By then Cutten was named president of Colgate and, eventually recruited Estabrooks to the Colgate faculty. Both Cutten and Estabrooks contributed in significant ways to the emerging "modern" theory of hypnosis. Estabrooks' last publication (1965) discussed the role of hypnosis in the treatment of academic under-achievement (Kihlstrom and Frischholz 2010, 87).

Another influential member of the Colgate faculty was William E. Edmonston (born 1931), who joined in 1964 at the invitation of Estabrooks. He became professor in the Department of Psychology and was chair of the psychology department from 1971 to 1975 and from 1978 to 1981. He was also the second editor of the *American Journal of Clinical Hypnosis* (AJCH: 1957–1968), following Erickson, the journal's founding editor. One of Edmonston's former students at Colgate, the psychologist John F. Kihlstrom and Edward J. Frischholz (editor of AJCH from 1995 to 2001), wrote about Edmonston:

> At the height of the new "golden age" of hypnosis, Edmonston con-vened a conference of hypnosis researchers, clinicians, and theorists under the auspices of the New York Academy of Sciences – the first time that distinguished institution had taken official note of hypno-sis (Edmonston, 1977c). On sabbatical as a Fulbright Scholar and Gastprofessor at the University of Erlangen-Nürnberg in Germany, Edmonston prepared a history of hypnotic induction techniques cov-ering a huge swath of territory from the sleep temples of ancient Egypt, Greece, and Rome to the Stanford and Harvard scales, the Creative Imagination Scale, and the Hypnotic Induction Profile (Edmonston, 1986). The book concludes with the prediction that the eyes – "the only naturally visible parts of the central nervous system" (p. 386) will prove to be the keys to understanding hypnosis and hypnotizability(Edmonston 2010, 83).
>
> (Kihlstrom and Frischholtz 2010, 87)

Another pioneer and major figure is John Goodrich (Jack) Watkins (1913–2012), Professor of Psychology and Director of Clinical Training at the University of Montana from 1964 to 1984. After earning a Ph.D. at Columbia University, Dr. Watkins began his academic and research career focused on psychology and the areas of hypnosis, dissociation, and multiple personalities.

In the 2009 presentation quoted in Chapter 3 (acceptance of the Dr. Bernauer W. Newton Award), he described his work during World War II at the Welch Convalescent Hospital in Daytona Beach, Florida, a 5,000-bed installation. At Welch he worked on the rehabilitation of "combat casualties from the Western Front, one half of whom were orthopedic and one half war neuroses." He developed hypnoanalytic techniques in the treatment of war neuroses and worked on issues related to the treatment of excessive sleepiness or the inability to sleep. With his wife Helen Watkins, he developed ego-state therapy which uses hypnosis to analyze underlying personalities.

Among the most fascinating portions of John (Jack) Watkins's presentation of 2009 was his summary of the beginning of America's formal professional organizations related to and promoting the use of hypnotism. Only direct quotes can convey the full flavor and so elegantly reflect their embryonic years:

> In 1949, 25 active hypnosis publishers in New York, led by Jerome Schneck and Milton Kline founded SCEH, the Society for Clinical and Experimental Hypnosis. Because of my book, "Hypnotherapy of War Neuroses" (Watkins, 1949), I was invited to be one of the "founding" members. Hypnosis at that time was not accepted as reputable in the professional circles of medical, psychological, dental, psychiatric or psychoanalytic, so the organization decided to set very high membership requirements: five years experience, accreditation by a medical or psychological specialty board like the American Board of Surgery, and actual publication. The result was most practitioners could not qualify for membership. Consequently, another society, the American Society of Clinical Hypnosis, ASCH, was founded by Milton Erickson and his associates, who had been giving three-day workshops on hypnosis, and opened its membership to general practitioners (Watkins, 1995).
>
> Almost immediately, the two societies battled for members, turf and status, seeking approval from the American Association for the Advancement of Science and the World Society of Mental Health, et al. Eventually, ASCH raised its requirements for membership, SCEH lowered theirs, and the two organizations competed for members on a comparable level. ASCH soon grew rapidly in membership, but had more difficulty securing papers for its journal, the *American Journal of Clinical Hypnosis*. SCEH had less difficulty getting scientific papers, but, with fewer members, had difficulty financing its journal, the *Journal of Clinical and Experimental Hypnosis* (Watkins 1995).
>
> (Kihlstrom and Frischholtz 2010, 83)

He continued his presentation by describing the beginnings of "The American Board of Hypnosis" (under the aegis of SCEH, with sub-boards in medicine, psychology, and dentistry, which "initially were boycotted by ASCH"). SCEH then organized an "International" society which quickly grew into ISCEH with 24 different national divisions. Finally, according to Dr. Watkins, Stanford University's Professor Ernest Hilgard, a past President of the American Psychological Association, and Erika Fromm, psychoanalyst and professor at the University of Chicago, "resolved the warring issues," and Dr. Hilgard became the first president of the International Society of Hypnosis (ISH), which replaced ISCEH.

Dr. Watkins is a past president of the Society for Psychological Hypnosis, Division 30 of the APA, of SCEH, and of the American Board of Psychological Hypnosis. Dr. Watkins was also a prolific writer of books and articles and, in 2005, co-authored with Arreed Franz Barabasz a revised edition of his earlier classic text (1987) "specifically intended to meet the current and emerging needs of a university graduate program to train psychologists and medical practitioners in the use of hypnosis."

Barabasz is also a past president of both SCEH and of the Society for Psychological Hypnosis, Division 30 of the APA. Dr. Barabasz earned his Ph.D. in Clinical and Human Experimental Psychology at the University of Canterbury, New Zealand, in 1981. He is a psychologist in practice and professor and director of the Hypnosis Laboratory at Washington State University and editor of the *International Journal of Clinical and Experimental Hypnosis.*

Another extraordinary resident of Montana was Bernauer W. "Fig" Newton, Ph.D. (1917–2001). In recognition of his many decades of significant contribution to the field of hypnosis, in 2008 the ASCH established the Dr. Bernauer W. Newton Fund to further "the growth of clinical hypnosis by recognizing and celebrating outstanding individuals in the field." In addition to the professional award, the Fund provides scholarships for students in the fields of health and medicine.

The inaugural recipient was Dr. Ernest L. Rossi, Ph.D. (born 1933) who included in his acceptance lecture a paean to three of his teachers: Bernauer "Fig" Newton, Milton H. Erickson, and David Cheek.[9] Dr. Rossi recalled first meeting with "Fig" Newton 45 years earlier (in 1962); Newton was then a consultant in clinical hypnosis at the Mount Sinai Hospital in Los Angeles, California.

> I could not help suppressing a grin the first time I saw him. He certainly was a brilliant man, and yes, his face really did give humorous fig-like impression, somehow! His "Fig-ness" was only emphasized when his eyes crinkled as he smiled broadly because in that very first moment of our meeting *he silently knew that I knew that he was smiling because I was smiling in astonishment about the appropriateness of his nickname "Fig."* I could not have known it at the time, but this smiling, silent, and simultaneous perception of each other's thoughts and evanescent emotional states was a succinct example of what would later be called "The Neuroscience Theory of Mind," which found evidence for the activity of "Mirror Neurons" as the basis of empathy in apes and man. Mirror neurons are now recognized as a source of the basic talents of the psychotherapist in general and practitioners of therapeutic hypnosis in particular.
>
> (Rossi and Rossi 2006)[10]

Erickson's "General Waking Trance" and States of Focused Attention

The American psychiatrist Milton Hyland Erickson, M.D. (1901–1980) was one of the leading users of medical hypnosis and – throughout a professional career that spanned more than 50 years – conducted extensive research on *suggestion* and *hypnosis*. He received his M.A. and M.D. degrees from the University of Wisconsin (1928), entered into a general internship at the Colorado General Hospital, and from 1929 to 1930, was Assistant Physician at the State Hospital for Mental Diseases in Howard, Rhode Island.

In addition to his medical practice, in 1957 he became one of the founders of the ASCH and served as its first President. He also established and was editor for the first ten years of the AJCH.

According to the Erickson Foundation, when he died on March 25th, 1980, at the age of 78:

> his seminars were booked through the end of that year and requests exceeded another year's scheduling. Dr. Erickson left a written legacy of more than 140 scholarly articles and five books on hypnosis which he co-authored.
>
> The Ericksonian approach departs from traditional hypnosis in a variety of ways. While the process of hypnosis has customarily been conceptualized as a matter of the therapist issuing standardized instructions to a passive patient, Ericksonian hypnosis stresses the importance of the interactive therapeutic relationship and purposeful engagement of the inner resources and experiential life of the subject. Dr. Erickson revolutionized the practice of hypnotherapy by coalescing numerous original concepts and patterns of communication into the field.
>
> . . . Although he was known as the world's leading hypnotherapist, Dr. Erickson used formal hypnosis in only one-fifth of his cases in clinical practice.[11]

The psychologist and psychoanalyst Dr. Rossi had a close working relationship with Dr. Erickson during the last eight years of Dr. Erickson's life, as a colleague, a co-author on several books, and, later, also as one of the editors of the 16-volume *Collected Works of Milton H. Erickson* published by the Erickson Foundation Press. The second teacher Dr. Rossi mentioned in his 2008 ASCH acceptance speech was Dr. Erickson. He described some of his personal recollections in a segment titled "Milton H. Erickson, My Second Teacher of Therapeutic Hypnosis: Heat, Work and 'The Burden of Responsibility in Effective Psychotherapy'." He highlighted Dr. Erickson's approach which, he underlined, was based on the essential need for the patient to work and work hard toward a favorable resolution, a *solution* to the problem. In Dr. Rossi's words:

Now I suddenly understood the significance of the little known and appreciated paper he had published two decades earlier on "The burden of responsibility in effective psychotherapy" (Erickson 1964/2008). There is something very simple, reassuring, and yet profoundly paradigm shaking about the nature of the therapeutic hypnosis in this brief six page paper. Erickson maintained that *therapeutic hypnosis is not relaxation, sleep, or a "miracle of healing"*! Erickson, after all, came from a hard working family of farmers. He recognized the burden and worth of hard work when he saw it! *Therapeutic hypnosis and effective psychotherapy involved hard work – intense inner activity on the part of the patient – not necessarily the therapist!*

. . .

Erickson believed effective psychotherapy was the result of the patient's intense inner activity not the therapist! It was another 10 years before I realized that the patient's intense creative inner activity and work was fundamentally a manifestation of what the molecular biologist called *"activity-dependent gene expression and brain plasticity"* (Rossi 2009).

Dr. Erickson's "general waking trance" theory has been described as a bridge between traditional therapeutic hypnosis and modern neuroscience-oriented psychotherapy as practiced today. In a 2009 interview Dr. Rossi elaborates on this. It is "one of Erickson's fundamental concepts which Erickson himself never wrote about," said Dr. Rossi, but which he "considers as a breakthrough in the evolution of his own thought and practice." When Dr. Erickson explains his concept of "general waking trance" he is, according to Dr. Rossi, "describing states of focused attention, intense expectancy, mental absorption, and response attentiveness." This response attentiveness "is a so-called 'naturalistic trance' because it engages the person's intense interest, motivation, and 'fixed attention' without the use of any formal hypnotic induction technique," adds Dr. Rossi. In summary:

I now believe this is the essence of Erickson's "naturalistic" and "utilization" approach to therapeutic hypnosis, which many excellent psychotherapists actually use without labeling it as such. I have proposed that Erickson's intense state of response attentiveness during the general waking trance evokes the three psychological experiences of novelty, enrichment, and exercise (both mental and physical) that neuroscientists now use to turn on activity-dependent gene expression and brain plasticity that are the molecular-genomic basis of memory, learning, consciousness, and behavior change.

Beyond his close work and personal relationship with Dr. Erickson (as summarized above), Dr. Rossi is a Jungian analyst who has written or co-authored a large number of professional books and papers on psycho-therapy, dreams psychobiology, and therapeutic hypnosis. In addition to new concepts of hypnosis, his conclusions rely to a great extent on the evolving fields of molecular genetics, neurobiology, psycho-neuroimmunology, and neuroendocrinology. His contributions have been recognized in numerous ways by the leading professional organizations in the fields of hypnosis and psychotherapy. It is within the context of such eminent professional background that he has offered the following thoughts in an interview with Michael Yapko, Ph.D., back in 1990:

> The average psychotherapist is profoundly behind the times. The genius of our age is not in psychotherapy. That genius took place in the 1900s with Freud and Jung. The genius of our age is the molecular biology of the gene. The genius of the 1920s and 1930s was quantum physics. But, the average psychotherapist is hopelessly behind the times from the point of view of modern biology.
>
> Another way of saying the same thing is that every hypnosis journal – the *American Journal of Clinical Hypnosis*, the *International Journal of Clinical and Experimental Hypnosis* – is hopelessly behind the times. They are not publishing the innovative research in hypnosis. The innovative research in hypnosis is being published by journals in neuroscience, but they don't use the word "hypnosis" written in the title of the paper they publish. They have titles like "Ritualized Relaxation and Lymphocyte Movement," and "Imagery and Moncyte Movement." They are tracing the effects of images and emotional states on white blood cells and molecules, right down to the genetic level.
>
> (Yapok 1990)

More than two centuries after Mesmer's experiments with and use of self-hypnosis we now have a wave of many credible and well-documented examples of the use of this technique for a variety of health-related purposes. Among the most fascinating is its use by the Swiss psychiatrist and ground-breaking, prize-winning hang-glider, balloonist, and glider pioneer, Dr. Bertrand Piccard (born 1958). Dr. Piccard is the son of Jacques Piccard (the undersea explorer) and grandson of Dr. Auguste Piccard (the world-famous balloonist). He has combined his medical background with his training in the use of hypnosis. Among his many (non-medical) accomplishments is becoming the European hang-glider aerobatics champion in 1985 and the first to complete the successful non-stop circumnavigation of the Earth in a balloon. With Brian Jones as a partner and supported by a team of specialists (including meteorologists on the ground), the two left Switzerland in *Breitling Orbiter 3*, a balloon less than 17 feet in diameter, and successfully covered a distance of 28,431 miles to reach Egypt less than 20 days later. For this accomplishment, on April 7, 1999, Dr. Piccard and Jones were awarded a $1 million prize at the National Air and Space Museum in Washington, D.C.

In 2003 Dr. Piccard teamed up with André Borschberg, a Swiss professional pilot, in an ambitious plan to circumnavigate the globe in a solar-powered aircraft. Since 2008 he and his partners have built Solar Impulse and completed several challenging night and intercontinental flights, including the one in 2013 when Dr. Piccard and Borschberg traversed the United States from California to New York City. Solar Impulse was the first "airplane of perpetual endurance, able to fly day and night on solar power, without a drop of fuel." Because of weight limitations, only one pilot was able to be on board during flight. Aside from the human endurance limits, the pilot was also faced with the constant need to guide the slowly flying and unusually light aircraft. Because of shifting winds and air currents, in essence there is hardly any time to nap, let alone sleep during the flight itself.[12]

To get some rest and yet stay awake as needed during these demanding round-the-clock solar-powered flights, Borschberg used a form of yoga meditation while Dr. Piccard relied on self-hypnosis. He has lectured and written extensively on this topic (http://www.solarimpulse.com/). During 2014, Dr. Piccard and his *Solar Impulse* team (which includes several hypnotherapists who assist him) successfully completed a 72-hour simulation, during which he used hypnotic techniques that were closely monitored. Based on the earlier technology, a second aircraft was built and *Solar Impulse 2* began its round-the-world solar flight – without fuel, entirely powered by the sun – during March, 2015. The single-seat carbon fiber aircraft had a wing span of 236 feet (longer than a Boeing 747), the weight of a family car, and four electric engines powered through 17,248 solar cells. During a total of 23 days of flight, *Solar Impulse 2* traveled 26,744 miles at a cruising speed of 28–34 mph, from Asia to North America, Europe, Africa, and the Middle East. This round-the-world flight was successfully completed on July 26, 2016.

In a short video posted on his website (http://www.solarimpulse.com/en/tag/Bertrand-Piccard#.VC25RZDD-Uk), Dr. Picccard elaborated that during the actual circumnavigation flight he would be limited to 20-minute naps that will only add up to a total of two to three hours of sleep every 24 hours. Therefore, it is important that he "fall quickly into deep sleep." His use of hypnotic techniques helped him "go faster into relaxation" and achieve deep sleep sooner than is normal without hypnosis. In addition, post-hypnotic suggestions allowed him to re-focus on his tasks rapidly after his naps.

Dr. Piccard explained the evolution of his ultimately successful approach (http://bertrandpiccard.com/medicine-hypnose?width=927). At first he "was looking for a way of solving the problem of sleep deprivation during his balloon expeditions." That led him to "a special interest in hypnosis" in which, eventually he found "not just a way

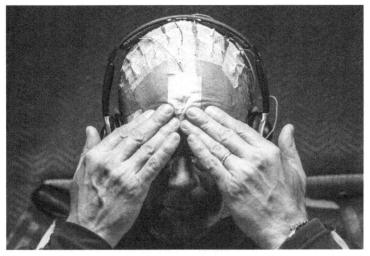

(a)

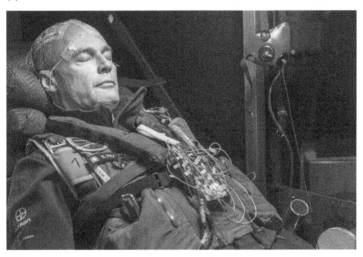

(b)

Figure 4.2 (a) and (b) two photographs of Dr. Bertrand Piccard practicing autohypnosis and the hypnotic techniques that he used while piloting Solar Impulse 2's around-the-world flight (2015 and 2016).
Dr. Piccard explained that during his longer flights of two and three days and nights he was limited to naps of not more than 20 minutes, for a total of two to three hours of sleep every 24 hours. Therefore it was important that he "fall quickly into deep sleep." He used hypnosis and autohypnosis to help him "go faster into relaxation and to achieve deep sleep sooner than it is normal without hypnosis." His training and preparation are further described at www.bertrandpiccard.com/medicine-hypnose. (Photos reproduced with permission from Solar Impulse. © Fred Merz, Solar Impulse, Rezo.ch © Jean Revillard/Rezo.ch/Solarimpulse).

of dealing with stress, fatigue and time taken to fall asleep, but more than that a genuine therapeutic procedure, centered on the use of inner resources and effective for treating patients suffering from anxiety, phobias, trauma or depression."

His training in hypnosis and self-hypnosis began in 1992:

> in anticipation of the first transatlantic balloon race that would consist of five days and five nights over the Atlantic in a tiny capsule. I use all these techniques when flying with Solar Impulse. In the case of resting periods, the method is to dissociate the head from the body. The body can regenerate into a very deep relaxation while keeping the brain alert enough to check the instruments and follow what happens during the flight.
>
> (www.solarimpulse.com/medicine-hypnose).

He continued this preperation in Europe with further training in the United States in Ericksonian hypnosis which he has now also "integrated . . . fully into his psychiatric practice."

During *Solar Impulse 2*'s stop in Phoenix (May 3–12, 2016), Dr. Piccard visited the Milton Erickson Foundation and paid tribute to "Milton Erickson, the inventor of modern hypnosis." He stated that "it was this hypnosis that I learned at the start of the 1990s in order to manage stress, fatigue and sleep for the transatlantic crossing by balloon" and, of course, later, with *Solar Impulse 2*. "I could not at that time have imagined," he added, "that Milton Erickson, probably one of the greatest pioneers of psychotherapy, would accompany me twice over the Pacific, by balloon and in a solar aeroplane!"

For many years in Switzerland Dr. Piccard also organized and led training seminars for doctors and psychologists. In his own words:

> With hypnosis, the patient immediately enters into a mechanism of change. This creates the confidence needed to induce him to accept what, until then, had remained unacceptable. A patient who has been depressed for several years and who, for a quarter of an hour or so, experiences a sensation of happiness and inner peace, is not cured. But he has seen proof that something within him is capable of changing. When a person who is suffering from chronic pain has the benefit of a general analgesia for a few minutes, he discovers that his pain is not necessarily a permanent fixture. If he can disconnect from the pain for a few moments, it means that relief could be made to last longer
>
> (Piccard 2013)

He continues, pointing out that "hypnosis is perhaps the branch of psychiatry that most resembles surgery" and explains that "you often have

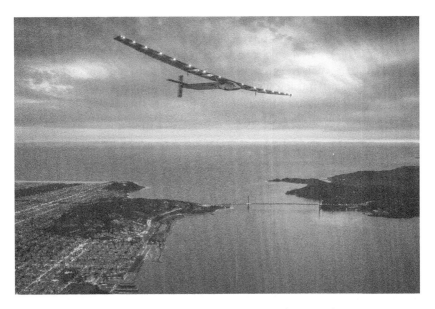

Figure 4.3 Solar Impulse 2 overflying San Francisco, after completing a 2,810-mile flight from Hawaii (April 23, 2016). Bertrand Piccard, M.D., was the pilot during the three days and two nights of the record-setting, entirely solar-powered flight. For the successful completion of this portion of Solar Impulse 2's round-the-world flight, Dr. Piccard relied on autohypnosis and other hypnotic techniques.

to open something up in order to repair it." He adds that "there's an important difference" in that "I do not act alone, but in collaboration with my patient." The patient is empowered, "he does the work – I just lend him company."

Finally, to give our readers a glimpse of the exciting future ahead for the science of hypnosis and its potential beneficial use in the treatment of sleep – as well as of many other – disorders, at this point the authors would like to highlight the work of J. Allan Hobson, M.D. (born 1933). Our last chapter will attempt to summarize our optimism and it seems appropriate to recognize many of the reasons given us by Dr. Hobson, a Professor of Psychiatry, Emeritus, Harvard Medical School and Professor, Department of Psychiatry, Beth Israel Deaconess Medical Center. He has offered wonderfully written, perspicacious insights into the many and somewhat parallel strands that propel this leap into our future. We are living through a period of almost impossible-to-describe or to fully comprehend advances in the study of the brain, of the states of sleep, dreaming, and hypnosis, and the differences between and among these states and the state of being awake.

Dr. Hobson is well known for his decades-long teaching and research while "quantifying mental events and correlating them with quantified brain events, with special reference to waking, sleeping and dreaming" (Hobson 2017). His books touch upon all of these topics and give us insights into recent research, discoveries, and the advances in understanding currently taking place, there for us to witness.

The remaining part of our work will focus on the use of hypnosis specifically in sleep medicine.

Notes

1 One of the best works on these intertwined strands is *Mesmerism and the End of the Enlightment in France,* by Robert Darnton, of Princeton and Harvard Universities, published in 1986 by Harvard University Press. Darnton examines mesmerism as a movement rather than a philosophy. Other excellent sources can be found in the 250+–volume Frank A. Pattie collection of books by and relating to Mesmer and the notions of "animal magnetism" that became associated with him. Of the 250 titles, about 50 date from the period 1746 to 1800, about 120 date from 1801 to 1900, and the balance consists of twentieth century studies, chiefly of Mesmer and his original tenets. Some of Mesmer's most important works (according to Robert Darnton in the *Dictionary of Scientific Biography*) are in the collection, including his *Précis historique des faits relatifs au magnétisme animal* (London, 1781) and his *Mesmerismus oder System der Wechselwirkungen, Theorie, und Anwendung des thierischen Magnetismus als die allegemine Heilkunde zur Erhaltung des Menschen,* edited by K.C. Wolfart (Berlin, 1814). The collection is named after the pioneering hypnosis researcher Frank A. Pattie (1901–1999), whose biography of Mesmer was published in 1994 by William Edmonston's boutique publishing company.

2 From: http://www.sciencepresse.qc.ca/blogue/2012/01/05/mesmer-magnetisme-animal, written by Ariel Fenster, January 5, 2012.

   « Écrit par Bailly, *Le rapport des commissaires chargés par le roi de l'examen du magnétisme animal* fut dévastateur. Il conclut qu'il n'y avait aucune évidence scientifique du phénomène et que les effets observés étaient le fruit de «l'imagination».

   « À la suite de la publication du rapport, la popularité de Mesmer s'évanouit. Il quitta Paris en 1785 pour retourner à Vienne d'où il était venu quelques années plus tôt. Aujourd'hui, on se souvient de Mesmer pour deux raisons: tout d'abord, Mesmer peut être considéré un précurseur de l'hypnotisme, une technique développée dans les années 1840 par le docteur écossais James Braid. Ce dernier s'est inspiré des expériences de Mesmer pour mettre au point les différentes formes de suggestion qui peuvent amener à l'état d'hypnose. Ensuite, le nom de Mesmer est à l'origine de l'expression de la langue anglaise *to mesmerize,* qui veut dire «fasciner», un terme bien en accord avec le personnage. »

3 The quotations from Benjamin Rush's *Medical Inquiries and Observations Upon the Diseases of the Mind* are as quoted in the Schneck (1978) *International Journal of Clinical and Experimetnal Hypnosis* article.

4 *Mesmerism* (G. Frankau, Introduction) London: Macdonald, 1948. (Originally published in 1779 in France, *Memoire sur la découverte du magnetism animal.* (*Dissertation on the discovery of animal magnetism.*)

5 In *Hypnotherapeutic Techniques*, 2nd edition, Chapter 1, page 11, Arreed Barabasz and John G. Watkins explain and provide further details of how ether and chloroform began to replace mesmerism:

> In Calcutta, hypnoanestheisa was for the first time practiced on a grand scale. True, scattered operations had been reported earlier in the United States, England, France, and Germany, but no one had before employed mesmerism for the wholesale relief of pain in hundreds of surgical cases, and no one has employed it so extensively since that time. Ether and chloroform were discovered. The more general applicability of chemoanesthesias, coupled with the unreliability of the mesmeric trance and the greater skill required for its use, soon settled the matter. However, at least one finding of Esdaile's has not been challenged to this day and is deserving of much further research. Although a high proportion of surgical cases died in surgery (or shortly afterward) of shock, almost none of those whose operations were conducted under mesmerism did so.

6 Alan A. Stone, M.D. (born 1929) is a professor of law and psychiatry at Harvard University. A graduate of Harvard University (1950) and Yale Medical School (1955), Professor Stone has been a Guggenheim Fellow, a Fellow at the Center for Advanced Study in Behavioral Sciences, and the Tanner Lecturer at Stanford University. He has been a film critic and reviewer for many years. Among his fields of interest are law and psychiatry, law and violence, and medical ethics (see: http://hls.harvard.edu/faculty/directory/10853/Stone). Among his books are *Movies and the Moral Adventure of Life* (MIT Press, 2007) and *Law, Psychiatry, and Morality: Essays and Analysis* (American Psychiatric Press, 1984).

During the past decades, the evolution of the use of medical hypnosis has attracted increasing scholarly scrutiny outside as well as within the United States. Among the many recent works in English are the following by Melvin Gravitz, J. Allan Hobson, C. H. Schenck et al., and Roberta Temes:

Hobson, J. Allan. 1988. *The Dreaming Brain: How the Brain Creates Both the Sense and Nonsense of Dreams.* New York: Basic Books Inc.

Hobson, J. Allan. 2002. *Dreaming An Introduction to the Science of Sleep.* Oxford: Oxford University Press.

Hobson, J. Allan. 2015. *Psychodynamic Neurology: Dreams, Consciousness, and Virtual Reality.* Boca Raton, Fl: CRC Press.

Hobson, J. Allan and Hellmut Wohl. 2005. *From Angels to Neurones: Art and The New Science of Dreaming.* Special Edition. Fidenza: Mattioli 1885.

Schneck, Jerome M. (Ed.) 1963. *Hypnosis in Modern Medicine*, 3rd ed. Springfield, Il: Charles C. Thomas.

Schenck, C. H., and M. Howell. 2013. "Spectrum of Rapid Eye Movement Sleep Disorder (Overlap Between Rapid Eye Movement Sleep Behavior Disorder and Other Parasomnia)." *Sleep and Biological Rhythms* 11(l): 27–34.

Schenck, C. H., J. L. Boyd, and M. W. Mahowald. 1997. "A Parasomnia Overlap Disorder Involving Sleepwalking, Sleep Terrors, and REM Sleep Behavior Disorder in 33 Polysomnographically Confirmed Cases." *Sleep* 20(11): 972–981.

Temes, Roberta. 1998. *Medical Hypnosis: An Introduction and Clinical Guide.* Medical Guides to Complementary and Alternative Medicine. New York: Churchill Livingstone.

7 Carl Stumpf's letter is included in the Gutenberg digitized files at http://www.gutenberg.org/files/40307/40307-h/40307-h.htm#page_247.

8 From: http://erickson-foundation.org/about/erickson/ as accessed on September 27, 2014, at 14:53.
9 From a transcript of Dr. Rossi's lecture, "The Psychosocial Genomics of Therapeutic Hypnosis, Psychotherapy, and Rehabilitation," published in a 2009 issue of the *American Journal of Clinical Hypnosis* and also published online 21 September 2011. (Please refer to the earlier, full citation.)
10 This excerpt and the following recollections are from *The Milton H. Erickson Foundation Newsletter*, Spring 2009, vol. 29, no. 1. "Interview with Ernest Lawrence Rossi, The Psychosocial Genomics of Art, Beauty, Truth and Psychotherapy: The Evolution of Ernest Lawrence Rossi's Thought and Practice," by Marilia Baker, Phoenix Institute of Ericksonian Therapy. Also, from the several Erickson Foundation Press publications, as mentioned in the text.
11 From the website of The Milton H. Erickson Foundation ("Biography of Milton H. Erickson" — https://www.erickson-foundation.org/biography / — and http://www.erickson-foundation.org/).
12 From the transcript of "My Solar-Powered Adventure," Dr. Piccard's presentation at TEDGlobal, filmed July 2009. From "Major Steps," http://www.solarimpulse.com/en/airplane/major-steps. *Solar Impulse*, December 31, 2011.
   A good summary of the genesis and development of the *Solar Impulse 2* project and Dr. Piccard's related use of hypnosis, autohypnosis, and hypnotic techniques can be found in "Solar Power: Solar Impulse 2 Circles the Earth," a full-page illustrated article in the *Frederick News-Post*, Frederick, Maryland, June 18, 2016. By Peter Janos Kurz: https://www.fredericknewspost.com/news/lifestyle/travel_and_outdoors/solar-power-solar-impulse-circles-the-earth/article_cca74022-8c77-588e-9ca1-ae3c611c4abe.html.

References

Barabasz, Arreed and John G. Watkins. 2005. *Hypnotherapeutic Techniques*, 2nd ed. New York: Brunner-Rutledge.

Bernheim, Hippolyte. 1885. *Suggestive Therapeutics: A Treatise on the Nature and Uses of Hypnotism*. New York: G. P. Putnam's Sons.

Binger, Carl A. L. 1968. "The Dreams of Benjamin Rush." *American Journal of Psychiatry* 125: 12; 1969: 67–73. Read as the Benjamin Rush Lecture on Psychiatric History at the 124th annual meeting of the American Psychiatric Association, Boston, Mass., May 13–17, 1968.

Braid, J. 1843. *Neurypnology, or the Rationale of Nervous Sleep*. London: J. Churchill.

Encyclopedia Britannica. 2005. Available online at: https://www.britannica.com/topic/animal-magnetism (accessed March 29, 2017).

Dessoir, M. 1888. *Bibliographie des modernen Hypnotismus* [*Bibliography of Modern Hypnotism*]. Berlin: Carl Dunchers Verlag.

Estabrooks, G.H. 1957. *Hypnotism*. New York: E.P. Dutton.

Gamwell, Lynn and Richard Wells. 1989. *Sigmund Freud and Art: His Personal Collection of Antiquities*, edited by Lynn Gamwell and Richard Wells. London: Harry N. Abrams, in association with the State University of New York and the Freud Museum, London.

Gravitz, Melvin. 1991. "Chapter 1: Early Theories of Hypnosis, A Clinical Perspective." In *Theories of Hypnosis. Current Models and Perspectives*, edited by Steven Jan Lynn and Judith W. Rhue. New York: Guilford Press.

Hobson, J. Allan. 1988. *The Dreaming Brain. How the Brain Creates Both the Sense and the Nonsense of Dreams*. New York: Basic Books.

Hobson, J. Allan. 2001. *The Dream Drugstore: Chemically Altered States of Consciousness*. Cambridge: The MIT Press.

Hobson, J. Allan. 2002. *Dreaming: An Introduction to the Science of Sleep*. Oxford: Oxford University Press.

Hobson, J. Allan. 2014. *Psychodynamic Neurology: Dreams, Consciousness, and Virtual Reality*. Boca Raton: CRC Press.

Hobson, J. Allan. 2017. "Faculty Profile Page." Available online at: https://sleep.med.harvard.edu/people/faculty/212/J+Allan+Hobson+MD (accessed April 2, 2017).

Hobson, J. Allan and Hellmut Wohl. 2005. *From Angels to Neurones: Art and The New Science of Dreaming*. Special Edition. Fidenza: Mattioli 1885.

James, William. 1890. *The Principles of Psychology*. Vols 1 and 2. New York: Henry Holt. From Vol. 53 of the 1964–1965 edition of the New York World's Fair Great Books of the Western World Collection, edited by Robert Maynard Hutchins. Encyclopaedia Britannica.

Jung, C. G. 1989. *Memories, Dreams, Reflections*. Revised ed. Recorded by Aniela Jaffe. Translated by Richard and Clara Winston. New York: Vintage Books.

Kihlstrom, J. F., and E. J. Frischholz. 2010. "William E. Edmonston, Jr.: Editor, 1968–1976." *American Journal of Clinical Hypnosis* 53 (2): 79–89.

Leitch, Alexander. 1978. *A Princeton Companion*. Available online at: http://etcweb.princeton.edu/CampusWWW/Companion/rush_benjamin.html (Rush, Benjamin), as found through http://etcweb.princeton.edu/CampusWWW/Companion/rush_benjamin.html .

Piccard, Bertrand. 2013. "Hypnosis as a Process Leading to Change." Available online at: www.bertrandpiccard.com.

Rosen, George. 1963. "Chapter 1: History of Medical Hypnosis: From Animal. Magnetism to Medical Hypnosis." In *Hypnosis in Modern Medicine*, 3rd ed., edited by Jerome M. Schneck. Springfield, Il: Charles C. Thomas.

Rossi, Ernest Lawrence. 2009. "The Psychosocial Genomics of Therapeutic, Psychotherapy, and Rehabilitation." *American Journal of Clinical Hypnosis* 51 (3): 281–298,

Rossi, E. and K. Rossi. 2006. "The Neuroscience of Observing Conscious and Mirror Neurons in Therapeutic Hypnosis." *American Journal of Clinical Hypnosis* 48:278–283.

Rush, Benjamin. 1830. *Medical Inquiries and Observation Upon the Diseases of the Mind*. Philadelphia: Grigg and Elliot.

Schneck, Jerome M. editor. 1953. *Hypnosis in Modern Medicine*, 1st ed. Springfield, Il: Charles C. Thomas.

Schneck, Jerome M. editor. 1963. *Hypnosis in Modern Medicine*, 3rd ed. Springfield, Il: Charles C. Thomas.

Schneck, Jerome M. 1978. "Benjamin Rush and Animal Magnetism, 1789 and 1812." *The International Journal of Clinical and Experimental Hypnosis* XXVI (1): 9–14.

Spanos, Nicholas P. and John J. Chaves. 1991. "Chapter 2: History and Historiography of Hypnosis." In *Theories of Hypnosis. Current Models and Perspectives*, edited by Steven Jan Lynn and Judith W. Rhue. New York: The Guilford Press.

Stone, Alan A. 2013. "Subject of Study." *Boston Review*, September 12. Available online at: http://bostonreview.net/film/stone-winocour-augustine-charcot (accessed March 25, 2017).

Sunnen, Gerard. 1998. "Chapter 2: What is Hypnosis?" In *Medical Hypnosis: An Introduction and Clinical Guide*, edited by Roberta Temes. New York: Churchill Livingstone.

Temes, Roberta. 1998. *Medical Hypnosis: An Introduction and Clinical Guide.* New York: Churchill Livingstone.

Watkins, J. 1994. "Historical Notes: The SCEH and ASCH, an Early Perspective." *Newsletter of the Milton H. Erickson Foundation* 14: 6.

Watkins, J. 1995. "Organization and Functioning of ISCEH." *The International Journal for Clinical and Experimental Hypnosis* XI (111): 332–341.

Watkins, J. 2009. "Hypnosis: Seventy Years of Amazement, and Still Don't Know What it is!" *American Journal of Clinical Hypnosis* 52: 2.

Yapok, Michael. 1990. "How I Became Ernie Rossi." An Interview with Ernest Rossi, Ph.D. Accessed through http://ernestrossi.com/interviews/Interview%20with%Rossi%20by%20Yapko.html.

5 The Selection and the Mechanics of Hypnotizing a Patient

Hypnotherapy may be utilized as part of the comprehensive evaluation and treatment of the patient's medical problem which is within the practitioner's scope of practice. Almost anyone who has a medical condition which has been shown to be amenable to hypnotherapeutic techniques might be considered for hypnotherapy. Hypnotherapy should not be utilized if the treatment may be better treated by non-hypnotic therapy.

Hypnosis is a natural phenomenon that can occur automatically in most people. Examples include daydreaming, or driving for several miles to your destination and having no memory of the intervening events – having been on automatic pilot. In hypnotherapy, the therapist assists the patient in obtaining the hypnotic state (trance) with various techniques, as discussed later in this chapter.

The ability to get into the hypnotic trance varies from person to person. Statistics vary, but, in general, 5% of people do not appear to be able to go into trance whereas 95% of people can get into at least a light trance. Fifty-five percent are able to get into a medium trance and 20% into a deep trance. The ability to get into trance is affected by chronological age, mental age, motivation, genetics, and by various environmental conditions.

Children are more easily hypnotized than adults. They are more suggestible and think more concretely. There is no significant difference between males and females as to hypnotic susceptibility (some therapists prefer the term *responsiveness*).

The relationship between genetics and hypnotizability (responsiveness) is still unclear but there appears to be a definite genetic contribution. Morgan (1973) studied hypnotic responsiveness of pairs of twins. Monozygotic twins were statistically more responsive than dizygotic twins. Raz, Fan, and Posner (2006) reported that polymorphism in the *COMT* (catechol-O-methyltransferase) gene was related to better hypnotizability. Subjects with the *COMT* gene combination valine/methionine were more highly suggestible than either methionine/methionine or valine/valine.

There are various clinical and standardized tests to evaluate the patient's potential to undergo hypnosis. Many clinicians feel that these tests do not reliably predict clinical outcomes for most medical disorders.

The standardized tests, however, are beneficial for evaluating which subjects to select for research purposes. Multiple factors contribute to the patient's response to hypnosis. The patient's expectations, beliefs, and attitudes are contributing factors.

The clinical techniques that can be utilized to indicate hypnotic susceptibility include *Spiegel's Eye-Roll Technique*, the *Arm-Drop Technique*, the *Postural-Sway Test* and others. Each has been shown to indicate the high possibility that the patient will be able to undergo hypnosis in the clinical setting.

Spiegel's Eye-Roll Technique

Dr. Spiegel (1972) performed the Eye-Roll Test on 2,000 consecutive cases in his clinical practice as part of preparation for a psychotherapeutic intervention which he reported in 1972. He indicated that the technique accurately predicted hypnotic trance capacity in approximately 75% of cases. The Eye-Roll Technique was one of the six items in the test of hypnotizability in *A Manual for Hypnotic Induction Profile* initially published in 1970 (Spiegel and Bridger 1970) which has subsequently undergone further revision. The technique generated controversy as to its accuracy, with proponents and detractors publishing articles over the ensuing years. The Eye-Roll Technique had significant test–retest reliability. It appears to show the capacity to undergo hypnotic trance but not necessarily hypnotizability. A patient may be able to get into a hypnotic trance but then not respond to the post-hypnotic suggestions with any alteration in thoughts or behavior. Nevertheless, it is quick to perform, taking approximately five seconds, and can be performed in the clinical environment.

The test procedure

1   Hold your head looking straight forward.
2   While holding your head in that position, look upward toward your eyebrows – now toward the top of your head (up-gaze).
3   While continuing to look upward, at the same time close your eyelids slowly (roll) (see Figure 5.1).
4   Now, open your eyes and let your eyes come back into focus.

The up-gaze and roll are scored on a zero-to-four scale. The amount of sclera visible between the lower eyelid and the lower edge of the cornea is the most practical measurement. A secondary measurement is upward movement of the cornea under the upper eyelid. Sometimes, during the up-gaze or roll, an internal squint occurs. The degree varies on a 1–3 scale (see Figure 5.2). This is a clinical "soft focus" observation which does not require discrete linear quantification with optical measurement instruments. The entire procedure can be done in about five seconds (Spiegel 1972, 26).

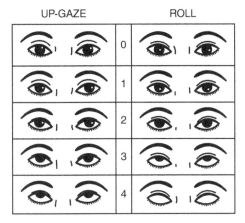

Figure 5.1 Eye-Roll Test for hypnotizability. (Reproduced from Herbert Spiegel. 1972. "An Eye-Roll Test for Hypnotizability." *American Journal of Clinical Hypnosis* 15, (1), with permission of the publisher, Taylor and Francis, www.tandfonline.com.)

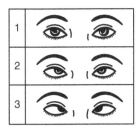

Figure 5.2 Eye-Roll Test (squint). (Reproduced from Herbert Spiegel. 1972. "An Eye-Roll Test for Hypnotizability." *American Journal of Clinical Hypnosis* 15, (1), with permission of the publisher, Taylor and Francis, www.tandfonline.com.)

There are numerous formal scales to evaluate hypnotic susceptibility. Although they are effective tools for evaluating hypnotic susceptibility for research purposes, they will not be described in detail since their relevance to clinical practice is questionable.

A number of the more common scales (listed in the References) include: Stanford Hypnotic Susceptibility Scale, Forms A and B (SHSS A and B; Weitzenhoffer and Hilgard 1959); Stanford Hypnotic Susceptibility Scale, Form C (SHSS C; Weitzenhoffer and Hilgard 1962); Stanford Profile Scales, I and II (SPS I and II; Weitzenhoffer and Hilgard 1967); Harvard Group Scale of Hypnotic Susceptibility (HGSHS; Shor and Orne 1962); Children's Hypnotic Susceptibility Scale (CHSS; London 1963); Stanford Hypnotic Clinical Scale for Children (SHCS-C; Morgan and Hilgard 1979).

This chapter's limited objective is to provide a brief overview. There are numerous books detailing the mechanics of hypnotizing a patient as well as describing various scales to evaluate the ability to be hypnotized and the potential depth of hypnosis. (Several are listed in our reference section.)

Before consideration is given to offering hypnosis as a means of therapy a complete medical history, sleep history, and physical examination should be performed as applicable to the therapist's practice. It should be emphasized that hypnosis should only be utilized as an additional tool for therapy within the scope of practice of the individual. Based on the clinical problem, if hypnosis is felt to be warranted as a method of treatment, a preliminary session with the patient is indicated to explain to the patient what is involved in hypnosis and to obtain a greater rapport with the patient by involving him or her in the therapeutic process. One of the most important aspects of the therapeutic hypnotic process is establishing a positive relationship with the patient. Although hypnosis is an altered state of consciousness, it is also an intensive interpersonal relationship between the patient and therapist.

To be effective therapists must inspire confidence that they are an expert at what they do and that the therapy will be successful, while at the same time they must avoid creating expectations that cannot be met.

During the initial interview it is important to encourage the patient to discuss his or her expectations concerning hypnosis and to describe any previous experience with hypnotic techniques. Any misconceptions of what hypnosis can or cannot do should be discussed and corrected at that time. Although patients cannot be made to do anything against their will or contrary to personal values, there is the possibility of the installation of false memories by an unethical therapist and certain areas of jurisprudence will not allow a person who has been hypnotized in the past to act as an expert witness. Patient misconceptions, such as the giving away of secrets and the loss of consciousness during hypnosis, need to be corrected.

Some practitioners ask the patient to read and to sign a treatment authorization and consent form. This can be a separate document or part of an overall consent signed by the patient at the time of the initial medical evaluation.

Various scales have been developed to measure both a patient's potential for hypnosis and the depth of hypnosis. However, hypnotizability scores do not necessarily correlate with treatment outcome. As a practical routine, after the evaluation noted above, the therapist proceeds with an induction with the assumption that the results will be successful.

There are many ways to induce the hypnotic trance – the state of hypnosis. A number of these will be briefly described. Other techniques can be found in Chapter 8. Some successful techniques for children are outlined in *Hypnosis and Hypnotherapy with Children* by Olness and Kohen (1996). There is no "best method" for helping the patient accomplish the hypnotic trance. It is of paramount importance that the therapist establish rapport with the patient and instill confidence that the therapist will be able to meet the patient's needs. The following is a brief overview.

Eye Fixation

The patient is asked to fixate on a point while sitting comfortably in a chair. The point should be elevated so that the eyes have to gaze somewhat upward in order to induce ocular fatigue. In a variation of this, the therapist holds an object, such as a pencil, just above the bridge of the nose. Verbalizations such as "your eyes are blinking and your eyelids are going to become heavier and heavier; they will want to close and not want to open" are timed with the patient's normal eye blinking. Typically the induction is felt to be successful when the eyes are firmly closed. However, induction may occur in some patients with the eyes still open.

Direct Stare

This is a technique for rapid induction. It requires an authoritarian approach and is rarely used in current hypnotherapy which utilizes a more passive approach to induction. A passive variation of the direct stare is at times utilized but is more difficult than the authoritarian approach. The patient typically would be sitting or lying down, but could be standing, with the therapist's head and eyes above those of the patient and in close proximity. The patient is commanded with a firm loud voice to look into the eyes of the therapist. Suggestions are made that the eyelids are becoming heavier, that they are shutting tightly and cannot open. The therapist may place his or her hand on the patient's shoulder or the top of the patient's head, holding it towards the therapist. If the patient's gaze turns aside s/he is told, "look at my eyes, but you can't, your eyes are fluttering and have shut, you cannot open them." Similar verbiage is repeated as needed. In the passive approach, the therapist demonstrates that s/he is sensitive to the patient's feelings and is kind and understanding. Looking into the therapist's eyes should elicit feelings of understanding and confidence that the patient can drift into hypnosis.

Coin Technique

A coin, no smaller than a quarter, is placed in the palm of the patient's hand with the suggestion that the hand will slowly turn and the coin will fall. Hearing the coin hit the floor will be the signal for the eyes to close and for the patient to become deeply relaxed. A variation of this is to place the coin between the thumb and first finger with the suggestion that the fingers will become tired and the coin will fall to the floor, which is a signal for the eyes to close by themselves. Another variation is to begin the induction with the patient's eyes closed and the coin placed in the patient's hand with the instruction to clasp it tightly. Suggestions are given for the hand to relax to the point when the coin falls to the floor, which will be the signal for immediate deep relaxation.

Postural-Sway Technique

This technique has been correlated with hypnotizability. The patient is asked to stand with heels and toes together. A soft, cushioned chair should be placed behind the patient. The patient is instructed to close the eyes and take several deep breaths. S/he is asked to imagine that the feet are hinged to the floor and that s/he is standing upright. It is suggested that the patient may feel unsteady but not to worry since "if" – or, it may be suggested, "when" – the patient falls the therapist will catch him or her. If the therapist is convinced that the "when" will be a success it should be used without hesitant instruction. As the swaying increases suggestions are repeated, "swaying forward, swaying backward," with the emphasis on backward. The depth of the trance can be estimated by whether the patient is limp, or attempts to catch him- or herself, at which time the therapist would put a hand behind the patient's back and ease the individual into the chair. As another option, the therapist can place a hands behind the subject's back just below the neck and the other near the upper front shoulder to give assurance to the patient that s/he will not fall; this verifies that the patient is indeed swaying. The patient's moves will just barely touch the therapist's hands.

Arm Drop Induction Method

The patient is asked to raise an arm so that the hand is slightly above the patient's head. S/he is then asked to stare at one of his or her fingers and the suggestion is made that as the patient stares at that finger the other fingers will tend to fade and the arm will begin to feel heavier and heavier. Repeated suggestions of heaviness are timed with movement of the arm. It is suggested that the patient will not go into a deep state of relaxation until the arm is all the way down. The arm is placed in a position such that gravity and fatigue will eventually cause it to move.

Another arm-lowering method is to ask the patient to stretch a hand straight out with the palm facing up and to imagine a heavy object, such as a dictionary or large rock, being placed in the hand. Suggestions for heaviness are given and that the hand will soon want to drift down; "just let it happen". Additional weight can be added as indicated. Suggestions for heaviness and movement should be timed to the actual movement of the arm.

Hand-Levitation Technique

The patient is instructed to place the hands comfortably on the thighs or the arm of the chair. The patient is asked to feel the warmth of his or her skin and the texture of the object s/he is touching. The patient is asked to imagine a string tied around the wrist with helium-filled balloons at the other end of the string, and to focus on the lightness of the balloons and how s/he may notice that "the hand" also begins to feel light. Further suggestions of lightness and movement are timed with slight movements of the finger or hand. Suggestions may be made that as the hand feels lighter and moves the rest of the body will relax.

There are many variations of this technique. The author suggests to the patient that as the hand drifts upward it feels that it is being drawn to the face like a magnet. As the hand touches the face it becomes heavy and drops back into the patient's lap.

Progressive Relaxation Techniques

The patient is asked to get into a comfortable position, generally sitting in a comfortable chair, although lying in a bed or couch is also an option. S/he is asked to focus on how specific muscle groups feel and then slightly to tense the muscle groups followed by relaxing them and to note the changes in sensation. Detailed lengthy suggestions may be utilized which are more specific to certain major muscle groups. Suggestions may be made that as you breathe in and breathe out you will automatically be more relaxed. The therapist gives instruction in a soft voice, accentuating the relaxation.

Deepening of the hypnotic state may occur rapidly or progress slowly depending on the induction technique and susceptibility of the patient. The deeper the trance state, the more likely that the suggestions made during the trance will be subsequently carried out. However, successful therapeutic suggestions can occur in light or medium hypnotic states. The success of hypnosis does not require that the patient reach a deep level of trance. Many patients will experience positive results while in their own mind they are still waiting to be hypnotized. The depth of hypnosis can be judged by the difficulty of the suggestion which the patient will accept. The induction techniques noted above, particularly when prolonged, can deepen the trance. Specific suggestions such as descending a stairway as you go deeper and deeper have been employed as has the use of a metronome. A metronome is set at approximately 60 bpm and the patient is told that relaxation will become deeper with each tick of the metronome. The words "deeper and relaxed" are reiterated to coincide with the metronome tick.

Once the patient has reached a desirable level of trance the "work" of the hypnotic suggestion will begin. Post-hypnotic suggestions (suggestions made during the hypnotic trance) are made concerning what activities are to be carried out after the termination of the hypnotic state (i.e., the treatment). Direct or indirect suggestions may be made. In general, indirect suggestions are more powerful. An excellent resource for suggestions can be found in Dr. D. Corydon Hammond's (1990) *Handbook of Hypnotic Suggestions and Metaphors.*

After the appropriate post-hypnotic suggestions have been made, steps are taken to "dehypnotize" the patient. The patient is informed that s/he will be awakened and all suggestions made during the trance which are not to be carried into the post-hypnotic state should be canceled. Post-hypnotic suggestions that are intended to remain are repeated. Suggestions are given that each time the patient undergoes hypnosis, s/he will do it quicker, better, and easier. The patient may also be given a specific signal to utilize in future sessions for more rapid re-induction. Prior to arousal from the trance suggestions are given for feelings of comfort that will continue on into the hours to come.

Following the hypnotherapeutic session it is valuable to discuss with the patient how s/he felt about it and ask for any suggestions for improving the process, including the induction technique. A second session may be held after this discussion or at a future date. Classically, an audio tape is made of the session that the patient is asked to practice. With the advance in electronics, a smartphone or other electronic device for recording and playback can be utilized.

Hypnosis is a valuable clinical tool that can be used to treat many medical conditions, including sleep problems. Like any tool, it is not effective for everyone. If utilized within the practitioner's scope of practice, experience, and competence, it has very few, if any, drawbacks.

References

Hammond, D. Corydon. ed. 1990. *Handbook of Hypnotic Suggstions and Metaphors.* New York: W. W. Norton.

London, P. 1963. *Children's Hypnotic Susceptibility Scale.* Palo Alto, Ca: Consulting Psychologists' Press.

Morgan, A. H. 1973. "The Heritability of Hypnotic Susceptibility in Twins." *Journal of Abnormal Psychology* 82: 55–61.

Morgan, A. H. and E. R. Hilgard. 1979. "The Stanford Hypnotic Clinical Scale for Children." *American Journal of Clinical Hypnosis* 21: 78–85.

Olness, Karen and Daniel P. Kohen. 1996. *Hypnosis and Hypnotherapy with Children,* 3rd ed. New York: The Guilford Press.

Raz, Amir, Jin Fan, and Michael. I. Posner. 2006. "Neuroimaging and Genetic Associations of Attentional and Hypnotic Processes." *Journal of Physiology Paris* 99: 483–491.

Shor, R. E. and E. C. Orne. 1962. *Harvard Group Scale of Hypnotic Susceptibility.* Palo Alto, Ca: Consulting Psychologists' Press.

Spiegel, Herbert. 1972. "An Eye-Roll Test for Hypnotizability." *American Journal of Clinical Hypnosis* 15 (1) (July): 25–28.

Spiegel, H. and A. A. Bridger. 1970. *A Manual for Hypnotic Induction Profile.* New York: Soni Medica.

Weitzenhoffer, A. M. and E. R. Hilgard. 1959. *Stanford Hypnotic Susceptibility Scale Forms A and B*. Palo Alto, Ca: Consulting Psychologists' Press.

Weitzenhoffer, A. M. and E. R. Hilgard. 1962. *Stanford Hypnotic Susceptibility Scale, Form C*. Palo Alto, Ca: Consulting Psychologists' Press.

Weitzenhoffer, A. M. and E. R. Hilgard. 1967. *Revised Stanford Profile Scales of Hypnotic Susceptibility, Forms I and II*. Palo Alto, Ca: Consulting Psychologists' Press.

6 A Brief History of Recent Developments in the Treatment of Sleep Disorders

Humans have always had an interest in sleep. With the advancement of scientific exploration, the evaluation and treatment of sleep disorders became possible. The clinical roots for the practice of sleep medicine date to the 1950s, as discussed in Chapter 2.

In addition to the seminal works of Kleitman, Aserinsky, and Dement, another important development was the discovery in the late 1950s of the suppression of muscle activity that takes place during rapid eye movement (REM) sleep. The renowned French sleep researcher Michel Jouvet observed that in the cat's REM sleep there was suppression of muscle activity during the electromyogram. We now take for granted the various stages of sleep, but it took years to put all the pieces in place.

The decade of the 1960s witnessed a rapid expansion of interest and research into the basic mechanisms and potential clinical applications of sleep. Numerous laboratories in the United States and abroad were involved in this important work. Doctors Ismet Karacan and Robert Williams of the University of Florida studied subjects at various ages in order to describe normal age-based sleep parameters. There was ongoing basic and clinical research with the development of tools for quantitative sleep analysis.

At the University of Florida I remember (WCK) many a night in the basement of the medical center monitoring monkeys with electrodes implanted in their brains. In order to help pay my way through medical school I worked as a sleep technologist for Doctors Karacan and Williams. This initiated my lifelong interest and excitement in the field of sleep medicine. In 1968 I published the first description of sleep parameters in two-year-old children and the association of dreaming with REM sleep in that age group in the *Journal of Pediatrics* (Kohler, Coddington, and Agnew 1968). (See Appendix A for complete article.) The research for that article was carried out in order to find normative data for two-year-olds. Under the mentorship of R. Dean Coddington I had evaluated twins, one with developmental delay, and had noticed that there was a change in REM percentage as the infant with developmental delay improved. We felt that REM sleep percentage could be a possible marker for psychological development. There were no normative data available and we undertook the two-year-old study to obtain that data.

A meeting of sleep researchers was held in 1960 for the purpose of adopting a standard scoring system for stages of sleep. A standard scoring system was not adopted at that time but the charter members agreed to meet annually to communicate their research findings. The Association for the Psychophysiological Study of Sleep (APSS) was formed in 1964. Concern continued as to the unreliability of the scoring that was utilized by various researchers. A committee was formed and in 1968 *A Manual of Standardized Terminology, Techniques and Scoring System for Sleep Stages of Human Subjects* was published, with Allen Rechtschaffen and Anthony Kales as the editors. The manual was intended to be utilized for evaluating research subjects, not for evaluating patients with sleep disorders. It became known as the "R and K manual" and was used by sleep researchers and clinicians as the ultimate standard for scoring sleep until 2007, when *The AASM* [American Academy of Sleep Medicine] *Manual for the Scoring of Sleep and Associated Events* was published. *The AASM Manual* was further refined in 2014 and continues to be considered a work in progress (Berry et al. 2014).

By 1975 sleep centers were examining patients and providing overnight sleep studies. A new organization was formed by leaders of the APSS, called the Association of Sleep Disorders Centers (ASDC). The Clinical Sleep Society (CSS) was formed in 1984 for individuals interested in the clinical aspects of sleep disorders. The ASDC-CSS was reorganized into the American Sleep Disorders Association in 1987 and the name was changed to the AASM in 1996. (For more information about the history of the development of sleep medicine in the United States, see Shepard et al. 2005.)

In 1964, William Dement and Stephen Mitchell established the first narcolepsy clinic at Stanford University, although it would be decades before sleep medicine itself would become an independent specialty.

One of the important steps in advancing the clinical field of sleep medicine was the recognition of sleep apnea in the mid-1960s and the subsequent development of treatment utilizing continuous positive airway pressure (CPAP) in the 1980s. The use of CPAP enabled the establishment of sleep medicine as an independent clinical practice. Previously, clinical practitioners interested in sleep medicine had to have an additional clinical practice, such as neurology or pulmonology, to be financially viable.

Sleep medicine was acknowledged as a distinct specialty by the Accreditation Council on Graduate Medical Education, which approved a Sleep Medicine fellowship program in 2004. In order to be an effective, viable specialty, continued basic research into sleep disorders and effective treatment needs to be carried out along with education of both the public and the medical profession.

Hypnosis has an important role to play in the treatment of sleep disorders. This role needs to be expanded and recognized through continued research and education.

A sample of sleep disorders that are currently being treated by sleep physicians is listed below. Those conditions that are currently being treated effectively, through the use of hypnosis and hypnotic techniques, will be discussed further and in greater detail in Chapter 7.

Apnea

Apnea by definition is cessation of airflow for more than 10 seconds at a time. The most common type of apnea is obstructive apnea, in which the airway is blocked off in spite of efforts to breathe. Anything that narrows the oropharynx or relaxes the pharyngeal musculature increases the likelihood that obstruction will occur. Enlarged tonsils in the child are a significant contributor to obstructive apnea. Tongue base enlargement and enlargement of the neck are frequently found in adults with sleep apnea. Central apnea occurs when the signals from the central nervous system to breathe are not present. Mixed apnea is a combination of central and obstructive apnea. If apnea occurs more than five times per hour for an adult or once per hour for a child, it is considered significant (Figure 6.1).

Hypopnea is a decrease in airflow followed by an arousal or decrease in oxygen saturation.[1] Both apnea and hypopnea can lead to significant morbidity. An apnea–hypopnea index for an adult of 5–15 is considered mild apnea, 15–30 moderate apnea, and above 30 severe apnea.

CLINICAL FEATURES	CHILDREN	ADULTS
Apnea Hypopnea Index	≥ 1	≥ 5
Peak Age	3-6 years	> 40 years
Gender	1:1 M:F (preadolescent	3:2 M:F
Snoring	+ (often continuous)	+
Witnessed apnea	+/–	+/–
Daytime Symptoms	Behavior problems decreased cognition EDS in minority	EDS
Associated Symptoms	Developental delay failure to thrive Minority	Complaints by partner
Obesity	Minority	Majority
Adenotonsillar Disease	Frequent	Uncommon

Figure 6.1 Comparison of sleep apnea in children and adults. EDS, excessive daytime sleepiness.

The apneas are recorded on the polysomnogram by use of nasal airflow monitors along with belts to measure chest and abdominal movement (see Figures 6.2–6.5, showing different types of apnea and obstructive hypopnea).

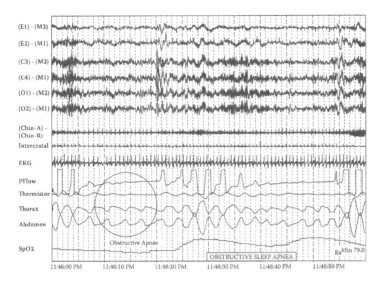

Figure 6.2 One-minute polysomnogram recording showing obstructive sleep apnea. Airflow has stopped with continued movement of thorax or abdomen.

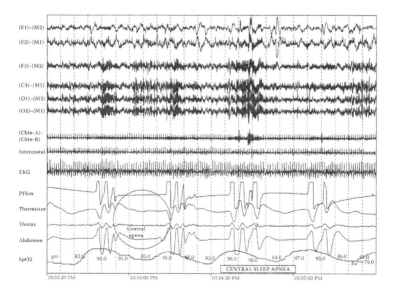

Figure 6.3 Two-minute polysomnogram recording showing central sleep apnea. Airflow has stopped and there is no movement of thorax or abdomen.

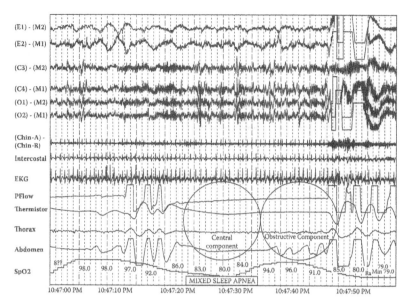

Figure 6.4 One-minute polysomnogram recording showing mixed sleep apnea. Initial lack of airflow and no movement of thorax and abdomen followed by movement in thorax and abdomen with continued lack of airflow.

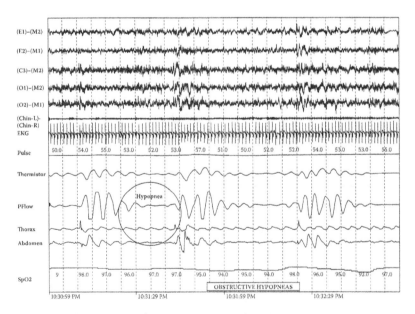

Figure 6.5 Two-minute polysomnogram recording showing obstructive hypopnea. Significant decrease in airflow with continued movement in thorax and abdomen with a 4% decrease in oxygen.

Apnea has been associated with the development of hypertension, heart attacks, stroke, dementia, elevated blood sugar, elevated cholesterol, erectile dysfunction, and an increase in accidents. When the apneic episode occurs, the only way to breathe again is to awaken. This disrupts the restorative function of sleep and can result in severe excessive daytime somnolence. One of my favorite jokes, and yet a truism, was a sign on the wall of a tire store that I noticed when I went to purchase a new set of tires. "I would like to die like my grandfather did . . . quietly, in his sleep, not yelling and screaming like the passengers in his car." Patients may awaken dozens of times per night with no memory of the awakening. Sleep apnea may be more severe in the supine position and in REM stage. During REM sleep the skeletal muscles are relatively paralyzed and there is an increase in oxygen consumption by the brain.

Prior to the development of CPAP the only effective treatment for severe obstructive sleep apnea syndrome (OSAS) was a tracheostomy. CPAP therapy is basically an air splint that keeps the airway open. A hose goes from a small air compressor to a mask on the face. There are three basic types of mask. One type goes over the nose, another goes over the nose and mouth, and a third type fits into the nostrils. It is crucial to find a comfortable mask in order for the patient to be compliant with CPAP use. Non-compliance with CPAP is a significant clinical problem, with compliance figures in general ranging from 50% to 75%. Hypnosis has the potential of improving this compliance, as discussed in Chapter 8.

CPAP is one type of positive airway pressure (PAP) therapy. Bilevel PAP (BPAP) devices have a constant pressure on inspiration with a reduced pressure during expiration. Adaptive servo ventilation (ASV) is a more recent development that has been found to be beneficial for both obstructive and central apneas. (ASV helps the patient take a breath if signals to breathe are not present.) Technology is advancing rapidly and there are various modifications of the current PAP therapy devices.

The surgical community explored various approaches to OSAS treatment with the development of the uvulopalatopharyngoplasty (UPPP), in 1981. Current surgery techniques for the treatment of OSAS include tracheostomy, nasal reconstruction, UPPP, both cold knife and laser, surgical tongue reduction, radiofrequency tongue reduction, genioglossus advancement-hyoid myotomy and suspension, and bimaxillary advancement or maxillary and mandibular osteotomy along with radiofrequency of the turbinates and palate. Most recently, hypoglossal nerve stimulation has been approved by the Food and Drug Administration for therapy.

Oral appliances for the treatment of sleep-disordered breathing have been developed. They enlarge the upper airway, stabilize the anterior position of the mandible, and advance the tongue or soft palate. They may also change upper-airway muscle activity. There are more than 50 patented devices available. To have maximum benefit, it is crucial to have a skilled practitioner evaluate and treat the patient with the proper device.

Currently hypnosis is not an effective treatment for sleep apnea, although it can help with CPAP compliance. It is conceivable that with further research hypnosis could become part of the therapeutic armamentarium for sleep apnea. Contributing to OSAS is a relaxation of the musculature in the oropharynx and tongue. Theoretically, post-hypnotic suggestion could improve neuromuscular tone.

Insomnia

Insomnia is a major sleep problem which most people have experienced at some point in their life. By definition, insomnia is difficulty getting to sleep or staying asleep, or non-restorative sleep. There are various types of insomnia with potential multiple causes. Insomnia may be primary or secondary to another health problem or medication. It may be acute, or chronic. It will be discussed further in Chapter 8. Ideally the cause of insomnia will be ascertained and treatment directed at the causal condition. Pharmaceutical companies have developed new compounds with the specific goal of treatment of insomnia. Benzodiazepines were first introduced in 1960. In the mid-1960s sleep laboratories were first utilized to evaluate sleeping pills. The relationship between pharmaceutical companies and sleep laboratories continues up to the present time. Drug companies continue to look for more effective, safer drugs to treat sleep disorders. However, medications have potential significant side-effects and are costly. Hypnosis offers an alternative therapy – without significant side-effects – that is cost-effective.

Parasomnia

Parasomnia is an experiential phenomenon that occurs around the time of sleep. These phenomena or undesirable events may occur on entering sleep, within sleep, or during arousal from sleep. They may occur in REM or non-REM sleep. REM parasomnias include nightmares, sleep paralysis, and REM sleep behavior disorder (including parasomnia overlap disorder). Non-REM parasomnias include sleepwalking, sleep terrors, and confusional arousals. Other parasomnias include sleep enuresis, sleep-related eating disorder, and sleep-related hallucinations. Medications have been utilized for parasomnias with mixed results. Hypnotherapy is an effective modality for treating parasomnias, as will be discussed further in Chapter 8.

Sleep-Related Movement Disorders

Sleep-related movement disorders include sleep-related rhythmic movement disorder, sleep-related bruxism, sleep-related leg cramps, periodic limb movement disorder, and restless-legs syndrome (Willis–Ekbom disease). Pharmaceutical companies continue to develop medications for these conditions. Hypnosis is a safe alternative effective therapy and will be further discussed in Chapter 8.

Hypnosis has an important role to play in the treatment of sleep disorders. As will be shown in the next chapter, hypnosis is already being used for the treatment of certain sleep disorders. With the addition of rapidly developing new technology and increasingly more effective techniques, our knowledge and experience with this valuable approach are expected to increase further. We hope and anticipate that hypnosis will be used far more extensively in the very near future.

Notes

1   Scoring of Hypopneas (Berry et al. 2014)
    AASM recommended definition

1A Score a respiratory event as a hypopnea if all of the following criteria are met:

    a   The peak signal excursions drop by ≥ 30% of pre-event baseline using nasal pressure (diagnostic study), Positive airway pressure (PAP) device flow (titration study), or an *alternative* hypopnea sensor (diagnostic study).

    b   The duration of the ≥30% drop in signal excursion is ≥10 seconds.

    c   There is a ≥3% oxygen desaturation from pre-event baseline or the event is associated with an arousal.

Or
AASM "acceptable" definition:

1B Score a respiratory event as a hypopnea if all of the following criteria are met:

    a   The peak signal excursions drop by ≥30% of pre-event baseline using-nasal pressure (diagnostic study), PAP device flow (titration study), oran *alternative* hypopnea sensor (diagnostic study).

    b   The duration of the ≥30% drop in signal excursion is ≥10 seconds.

    c   There is a ≥4% oxygen desaturation from pre-event baseline.

References

American Academy of Sleep Medicine (AASM) 2007. *Manual for the Scoring of Sleep and Associated Events: Rules, Terminology and Technical Specifications.* Darien, Il: American Academy of Sleep Medicine.

Berry, R. B., R. Brooks, C. E. Gamaldo, S. M. Harding, R. M. Lloyd, C. L. Marcus, and B. V. Vaughn for the American Academy of Sleep Medicine. 2014. *The AASM Manual for the Scoring of Sleep and Associated Events: Rules, Terminology and Technical Specifications.* Version 2.1. Darien, Il: American Academy of Sleep Medicine.

Kohler, William C., R. Dean Coddington, and H.W. Agnew, Jr. 1968. "Sleep Patterns in 2-Year-Old Children." *Journal of Pediatrics* 72 (2): 228–233.

Rechtschaffen, Allen and Anthony Kales (eds.) 1968. *A Manual of Standardized Terminology, Techniques and Scoring System for Sleep Stages of Human Subjects*. Washington, D.C.: U.S. Government Printing Office.

Shepard, John W., Daniel J. Buysee, Andrew L. Chesson, Jr., William C. Dement, Rochelle Goldberg, Christian Guilleminault, Cameron D. Harris, Conrad Iber, Emmanuel Mignot, Merrill M. Mitler, Kent E. Moore, Barbara A. Phillips, Stuart F. Quan, Richard S. Rosenberg, Thomas Roth, Helmut S. Schmidt, Michael H. Silber, James K. Walsh, and David P. White. 2005. "History of the Development of Sleep Medicine in the United States." *Journal of Clinical Sleep Medicine* 1 (1): 61–79.

7 The Successful Use of Hypnotic Techniques in the Management of a Dozen Sleep Disorders

As stated earlier, the use of hypnosis and hypnotic techniques can be very effective in the treatment of certain specific – although not all – sleep disorders. Its use should always be after proper medical evaluation by a properly trained professional who has decided that it was an appropriate form of treatment. This chapter will focus on listing a dozen sleep disorders which have been treated effectively through the use of hypnosis and hypnotic techniques.

Insomnia

A patient's common dilemma:

> Lying in bed, staring at the ceiling and a mind that won't shut off. Tomorrow is an important day. I know I need a good night's sleep to be alert. I've tried suggestions from friends and over-the-counter medications without help. What else can I do?

Insomnia has been defined as difficulty getting to sleep, staying asleep, or non-restorative sleep. It can be a disorder in itself or a symptom of another disorder – either medical or psychiatric. The incidence of insomnia varies depending on how it is defined; however, it is thought that possibly one-third of all Americans are affected by insomnia in one form or another.

The American Academy of Sleep Medicine in its *International Classification of Sleep Disorders* (3rd edition, 2014) defines insomnia as "a persistent difficulty with sleep initiation, duration, consolidation, or quality that occurs despite adequate opportunity and circumstances for sleep, and results in some form of daytime impairment."

It is common in the United States but even more prevalent in other areas of the world; it may be acute or chronic, and may occur at any age and in either sex, although prevalence increases in females and with age.

Insomnia affects not only the person involved but also the family and, indeed, society in general. People with insomnia miss a greater number of work days and are at increased risk for workplace accidents and errors. Healthcare costs for insurers are higher since people with insomnia use their physicians more often, are hospitalized more often, and have greater rates of disability and accidents. Insomnia has also been associated with depression and chronic pain.

If possible, the potential cause of insomnia should be established before treatment is initiated. Underlying psychiatric and medical conditions (such as depression, anxiety, asthma, pain, and hyperthyroidism) can lead to insomnia. Other sleep disorders such as sleep-disordered breathing and periodic limb movement disorder can also cause insomnia. Certain medical conditions such as hypertension, chronic pain, diabetes, coronary artery disease, cancer, and arthritis have been noted to commonly co-occur with insomnia.

Treatment of insomnia should be directed at the underlying cause. Most patients with insomnia do not seek treatment. When treatment does occur, most patients resort to over-the-counter remedies rather than seeking professional help. However, the physician has available both pharmacologic and non-pharmacologic treatment options. Hypnotic medications are available as well as behavioral approaches. Hypnotic medication has been shown to be beneficial in the short term, whereas behavioral intervention has been proven to have long-term efficacy.

As with any successful intervention, the cooperation of the patient is paramount. Biofeedback, relaxation training, aromatherapy, white noise, and adjusting the environment have been utilized to improve sleep. Studies have shown that cognitive behavioral therapy for insomnia (CBT-I) has proven effectiveness in treating insomnia. CBT-I includes:

- *sleep restriction:* restricting the time in bed to the actual sleep time and gradually increasing this as optimal sleep duration is achieved;
- *stimulus control:* reinforcing conditions that associate the bedroom with sleep and establishing a consistent bedtime and wake-up time;
- *relaxation training:* relaxation procedures to reduce muscle tension and intrusive thoughts;
- *cognitive therapy:* reframing faulty beliefs about insomnia and its daytime consequences;
- *education in sleep hygiene:* recommendations about noise levels, light, temperature, diet, and exercise.

CBT-I is time consuming for the practitioner and not many practitioners are trained in it. Fortunately, more education programs for the practitioner are becoming available. There are also internet-based providers of CBT-I which have been researched and validated.

Hypnosis, with its proven efficacy in improving anxiety and stress, is an ideal therapeutic intervention for many cases of insomnia. Before contemplating the use of hypnosis to treat the insomnia in a particular patient, a thorough medical and sleep history and a physical examination should be carried out to determine the potential causes of the insomnia.

A sleep diary should be maintained recording:

- the time of going to bed;
- estimation of length of time it took to fall asleep;
- the number of awakenings during the night;
- how long it took to get back to sleep;
- the time of final awakening in the morning;
- any naps;
- any associated activity that might influence sleep, such as alcohol, caffeine, or exercise close to bedtime;
- the total number of hours of sleep as well as its quality.

Hypnosis should be utilized in association with other behavioral techniques to improve the insomnia.

There are many good books about insomnia and its treatment, although very few mention hypnosis as a major and effective form of treatment. There are, however, numerous journal articles which have shown the efficacy of hypnotic techniques in treating insomnia. Several are summarized below.

Anderson, Dalton, and Basker (1979) reported on a trial comparing the treatment of insomnia with placebo, nitrazepam (Mogadon), and hypnosis. Included were 16 females and two males aged 29–60 who had had insomnia for at least three months prior to the trial. The types of insomnia varied, as did the hypnotic induction and deepening techniques. Although not specifically mentioned, it appeared that at least five different hypnotists were involved in the trial. During weeks one to four a double-blind trial of Mogadon and placebo was also carried out. Starting at week five all patients were instructed in the use of autohypnosis for insomnia. Details of the various hypnotic techniques were not given. It was stipulated that at least four sessions of treatment with autohypnosis would be carried out. Subjects continued using either Mogadon or placebo in addition to the autohypnosis until the end of week 8, at which time autohypnosis was utilized alone for an additional two weeks. Neither doctor nor patient knew whether they were utilizing Mogadon or placebo. Autohypnosis reduced the time taken to fall asleep and more patients had a normal night's sleep when utilizing autohypnosis alone than when they received placebo or Mogadon.

Bauer and McCanne (1980) reported on two cases of insomnia treated with short-term hypnotherapy. Patient One was a 45-year-old female with severe chronic insomnia dating back to her early 20s. Her sleep was restless, she slept between three and six hours per night, and was on medication for the insomnia. Case Two was a 27-year-old female with sleep disturbances for the past ten years which had become progressively worse.

She reported that at times she did not sleep at all but generally obtained between two and four hours of sleep per night. She was using medication for insomnia that appeared to have minimal effect. After an initial psychological evaluation and sleep history, the two patients were told that hypnosis had been successful with others for their insomnia and there was a good probability that it would be beneficial to them. They were to keep a record of their sleep and return in a week – at which time they were told they would be taught a technique that would allow them to fall asleep quickly. They were hypnotized utilizing a progressive relaxation induction with visual imagery. They were told:

> "to imagine themselves at a blackboard with a piece of chalk and an eraser, and they were asked to draw a circle on the blackboard and to write the number 100 inside the circle. It was suggested that they take the eraser, put it in the center of the circle and begin erasing the number slowly, by going in a counterclockwise circular motion, being very careful not to erase the outside edge of the circle."
>
> (Bauer and McCanne 1980)

They were told to write in script to the right of the circle the words "Deep Sleep." They were then instructed to go back to the circle and "write the number 99, erase it as previously instructed and then very carefully write over the words 'Deep Sleep', making sure that there were no double lines." They were told to repeat this procedure by subtracting one number at a time until they were asleep. It was emphasized that they should follow the procedure exactly but that they could proceed at a pace that was comfortable for them. At their two-week follow-up both patients reported good results and both had discontinued the sleep medication. At one-year follow-up both reported that they had "maintained relatively undisturbed sleeping patterns" (Bauer and McCanne 1980, 2–3).

Cochrane (1989) reported on the use of indirect hypnotic suggestion to improve insomnia while also addressing a patient's anxiety. The patient was a 44-year-old male with evidence of a generalized anxiety disorder. He was unable to sleep more than three to four hours per night. In Session One he described himself as an executive warrior, so hypnotic metaphors about soldiers were utilized.

> soldiers in Vietnam who, on the field of battle, understood that it was not safe to sleep deeply with the constant threat of the enemy nearby. It was suggested that when the war is over, it takes them a little time to realize that it is now alright to enjoy the pleasures and benefits of deep and restful sleep.

It was suggested that the patient's unconscious mind would utilize the tale in a healthy manner. The patient called the therapist five days later and reported that he was sleeping longer and deeper but requested another appointment. He now had concerns about his marriage and quality of life. Another hypnotherapy session was held with indirect suggestions focused on the above concerns. Follow-up contacts at nine months and two years revealed that the patient was sleeping between six and seven hours per night and in general was doing well (Cochrane 1989, 200–201).

Stanton (1989) studied 45 patients with insomnia. Nineteen males and 26 females participated in the project. They were divided into three groups for therapeutic intervention: hypnotic relaxation, stimulus control, and placebo. Sleep diaries and self-reports were utilized to measure the subjective complaints of insomnia. The subjects were to complete the diary on awakening every morning and mail it daily. Hypnotic relaxation was performed with visual imagery induction for Group One. Stimulus control instructions were given to the second group. The placebo group was given instruction in routine pre-sleep activities. The three groups underwent four weekly 30-minute sessions. Comparison of the three groups at the end of week four and at the three-month follow-up revealed a statistically significant difference between the groups: the hypnotic relaxation group had a significantly improved sleep-onset latency compared to the other two groups. The author concluded: "hypnotic relaxation is an approach to the treatment of sleep onset insomnia worthy of wider use" (Stanton 1989, 67).

Becker (1993) offered treatment with hypnotherapy to 22 consecutive patients with difficulty initiating and/or maintaining sleep. Six of these patients chose to try hypnotherapy and in preparation completed seven or more days of a sleep diary. These patients then underwent a thorough evaluation of their sleep complaints, medical history, and psychiatric assessment. Physical examination and additional testing were performed as indicated. All six subjects were diagnosed as having psychophysiological insomnia based on *International Classification of Sleep Disorders* criteria (American Academy of Sleep Medicine 2014). The initial session consisted of a discussion of hypnosis, the benefits of relaxation, and recommendations for deep sound sleep. A two-hour hypnotic induction session was performed. A second session of about one-and-one-half hours was held within three to seven days. Hypnotherapy was performed utilizing a modification of the technique of Bauer and McCanne, described above. Instruction with progressive muscular relaxation was given. Weekly sessions were held three more times. The session length depended on the improvement or lack thereof which had occurred. Three of the subjects showed significant improvement in their sleep after three sessions of hypnotherapy. This improvement continued in follow-up at eight and ten months.

Anbar and Slothower (2006) reported on the use of hypnotherapy in 84 pediatric patients who had difficulty falling asleep for more than 30 minutes at least once a week or who had frequent nighttime awakenings.

Ages ranged from seven to 17 years, with the duration of insomnia six months to five years. Assessment as to the effectiveness of the hypnotherapy was based on the patient's subjective reports. An initial hypnotherapy session was held for 15–60 minutes. At this time hypnosis was described and several induction techniques were demonstrated. Progressive relaxation as well as imagery of a favorite place were employed in addition to specific imagery intended to encourage sleep. The patients were asked to practice self-hypnosis at bedtime for at least two weeks and then on an "as needed" basis. Nine of the patients were lost to follow-up after this first session. If the insomnia was not resolved a second session was offered which provided additional instruction on gaining insight into potential stressors as well as education in sleep hygiene as indicated. The self-reported reasons for the insomnia included bedtime fears, stress over academic and family issues, difficulty with peers, environmental distraction, worries over the patient's own health, and early childhood abuse. The report indicated that in the majority of patients the insomnia resolved after one or two sessions. The report suggested that some of the improvement could be attributed to the effects of reducing physiological arousal, developing new thought patterns, and generating insight into the causes of their insomnia.

These cases point out how hypnosis can be successfully utilized to improve insomnia. Hypnotic techniques varied and were modified appropriately for developmental age. Direct and indirect suggestions can be utilized. Indirect suggestions are helpful in avoiding potential resistance. Many patients report that they are unable to "turn the mind off" – inhibiting them from going to sleep. Hypnosis can result in the reduction of physiological arousal as well as focusing their attention on suggested internal stimuli inhibiting them from the previously disrupting cognitive function. Therapeutic strategies are unique to each individual and should be utilized in conjunction with other therapies to improve insomnia. Hypnosis may not only improve the insomnia but also have a positive effect on other stress-producing situations which may be present.

Somnambulism

Somnambulism (sleepwalking) is a common parasomnia occurring in slow-wave non-rapid eye movement (NREM) sleep, generally during the first third of the night. It is considered a disorder of arousal. The underlying etiology is unclear. It has been associated with disordered breathing, including obstructive sleep apnea and upper resistance syndrome, restless-legs syndrome (Willis–Ekbom disease), periodic limb movement disorder, thyrotoxicosis, head injury, migraine, stroke, insufficient sleep, and certain medications. Zolpidem (Ambien) in particular has achieved notoriety for its effect on causing complex sleepwalking episodes such as driving a car. The first author had a patient who was using zolpidem who ended up at a gas station many miles from her home in her pajamas, not knowing how she got there.

Environmental stressors and anxiety may precipitate sleepwalking. Sleepwalking can occur at any age. In children it may begin as soon as the child can walk and commonly co-occurs with sleeptalking and night terrors. In childhood sleepwalking may occur in as many as 17% of children, with up to 25% continuing into adulthood. It has been estimated that up to 4% of adults sleepwalk.

There is a genetic component in some cases of sleepwalking, with rate of sleepwalking increasing in relationship to the number of affected parents.

Sleepwalking is usually benign but can be associated with violent behavior with injury to the patient or others in the environment. Inappropriate behavior may occur during the sleepwalking episodes, such as urinating on the wall or in the refrigerator, moving furniture, leaving the house, or climbing out the window. Sleepwalkers have been severely injured or killed by walking into traffic or falling out of a second-story window. The sleepwalker has little, if any, memory of the episodes. S/he may spontaneously return to bed or the episodes may end in unusual places. The patient's eyes are usually open with a glassy stare.

A variant of sleepwalking is nocturnal eating, during which the sleepwalker eats without being aware of this. Gaining weight while dieting, finding crumbs in the bed, and finding food left on the counter may be the only signs that nocturnal eating with sleepwalking has occurred. More dangerous activity may occur, such as a self-inflicted knife injury or accidentally setting the house on fire.

Sleepwalkers should gently be encouraged to go back to bed. They should not be forcefully aroused. Attempting to awaken them may cause them to strike out, potentially injuring a helper.

Infrequent and mild sleepwalking requires no intervention other than protecting the environment: removing dangerous objects from the room, locking doors and windows, and asking the patient to sleep on the ground floor. When the sleepwalking is severe active intervention is indicated.

As with any medical condition, a complete evaluation should be obtained in order to attempt to ascertain the underlying cause. Sleepwalking should be differentiated from other conditions that may look like it, such as complicated sleep terrors, REM sleep behavior disorder (RBD) and sleep-related epilepsy. Treatment should be directed at the causative factor or factors. Anticipatory awakening has been effective in some cases. The patient is awakened for at least five minutes approximately 30 minutes before the sleepwalking episode is anticipated.

Psychotherapy and pharmacotherapy have been utilized when no specific associated factor was ascertained. Drug therapy has included benzodiazepines such as clonazepam, diazepam, triazolam, flurazepam, and antidepressants. Carbamazepine and valproic acid have also been utilized.

Hypnosis has been utilized with success in treating parasomnias, including sleepwalking. Single cases and cases with a small number of patients treated with hypnosis have been reported along with the report of a single-blind crossover study. Reid (1975) reported on 12 military trainees with severe sleepwalking to the degree that they were facing honorable discharge. After indepth interviews by the author they were offered treatment for the sleepwalking or they could proceed with an honorable discharge. Six of the trainees desired treatment with hypnosis for their sleepwalking. They were told there would be no direct suggestions, only learnable methods of control, and that the sleepwalking should be considered to be occurring within a trance comparable to the trances experienced in the therapist's office and that they would learn a signal to alert them from the trance. The author indicated that the above concept was taken from a report by Dillahunt (1971), including the arousal cue which occurred when the patient placed the feet flat upon the floor.

The initial session included teaching the patient to relax and obtaining a light trance using the "point-concentration method" of induction (the patient is asked to pick a point straight out and stare at it with the suggestion that the eyes would become heavier and heavier and would want to close). He also used the "descending stairway deepening technique" (the patient is asked to imagine slowly walking down a stairway with visualization and feeling of the railings and carpet). The sessions were subsequently held twice a week for three weeks and lasted half an hour each. Four of the subjects reported complete alleviation of their sleepwalking and were able to complete their military training without incident.

Reid, Ahmed, and Levie (1981) reported the use of hypnosis in 11 subjects utilizing a modified single-blind crossover procedure. The subjects were initially rated for the quality of sleepwalking symptoms and the discomfort derived from them. Most of the subjects had been sleepwalking since childhood and were regularly sleepwalking at least twice a week. Subjects were assigned either to the active group that underwent hypnosis or the group where only suggestion was utilized. Two half-hour sessions per week were held over three weeks, with the results rated by a research assistant who did not know to which group the subjects were assigned. An additional three weeks of treatment were recommended with the opportunity for the subjects to switch groups. In the active group, a light trance was induced using the "point-concentration method" of induction and deepening with the "descending staircase." This active group was hypnotized with legs extended and feet resting on a footstool. While in the trance, it was explained to the subjects that sleepwalking occurs in a kind of trance and that when their feet are flat on the floor they would immediately become alert and awake no matter how deep a trance they were in. Suggestions for encouragement and well-being were also made. At the end of the session they were asked to place their feet on the floor and observe how rapidly the trance state disappeared. The suggestion group underwent the same induction and deepening method. Once in the trance suggestions were made for "improvement" and "whatever the cause of your sleepwalking, its needs have passed" (Reid, Ahmed, and Levie 1981, 33). Seven of seven subjects in the active group improved by the end of three weeks, with several being symptom-free. In the suggestion group two of four subjects improved dramatically. At a three-month follow-up one of the active group subjects had a return of symptoms but improved again with treatment with diazepam. The two subjects who improved in the suggestion group remained stable. Follow-up at one year revealed improvement had continued for the nine subjects.

Gutnik and Reid (1982) reviewed the treatment of sleepwalking, including hypnosis, and stated that 50% or more of the cases that they treated with hypnosis had been successful utilizing a "specialized form of hypnosis." The basic technique was the one described in the two reports listed previously. The hypnotic sessions were held with the patient's feet resting on a footstool. The authors emphasized that the learning paradigm consisted of two principles. One: "Your sleepwalking occurs in a kind of trance, a somnambulistic trance, much like the one you experience here in the office." Two:

> When your feet are flat on the floor, you will find that you immediately become alert and awake, no matter how deep the trance, no matter how deep your sleep. You will not be able to stay in trance, you will not be able to stay asleep, when your feet are on the floor.
>
> (Gutnik and Reid 1982, 311)

Hurwitz et al. (1991) reported on 27 patients successfully treated with hypnosis. Eight had primary sleepwalking, four primary sleep terrors, and 15 had combined conditions. The hypnotic trance was induced utilizing the:

> technique of suggesting eye closure during upward gaze and subsequent relaxation and sensation of floating. Then, patients were asked to visualize themselves in a pleasant, comfortable scene where they could find an imaginary screen on which to watch a time-lapse film of themselves sleeping quietly and peacefully through an entire night.

Suggestions were made for anxiety reduction and security along with "restful sleep with minimal movement." The session lasted approximately 20 minutes and was recorded on an audio cassette which the patient was to practice twice daily, including practice just before retiring. One of the authors treated six of the patients and another author treated 21. One to six sessions were held, with 17 patients having had only one treatment session prior to the follow-up assessment. Six of these stopped hypnosis, claiming that it was of no benefit. Only three patients had more than two sessions. The patients were contacted between six and 63 months after treatment through telephone by a nurse not involved in the therapy. Six patients reported very much improvement, 14 much improvement, and seven said that the symptoms were unchanged.

Kohen, Mahowald, and Rosen (1992) reported the successful use of hypnosis in four children with severe NREM disorders of arousal. Three of the children were age eight at the time of evaluation and one was age 11. Two of the children had sleep terrors, two had confusional arousals, and all of them had episodes of sleepwalking. After a thorough evaluation, including a polysomnogram (PSG), the children were given imipramine at bedtime in an attempt to control the arousals. Instruction was given in "self-regulation techniques using relaxation and mental imagery (RMI) (self hypnosis)" (Kohen, Mahowald, and Rosen 1992, 235). Once this was accomplished the medication was tapered and discontinued.

At the time of the first visit, which lasted approximately one hour, the parent and child were educated about night terrors. Suggestions for empowerment over the troublesome night terrors were provided. Each child was taught self-hypnosis during the last 20–30 minutes of the session. The induction reportedly was accomplished easily with:

> just close your eyes and have a wonderful daydream about some-
> thing you enjoy doing very much . . . with emphasis on options for
> imagery based on his/her personal favorite activities. I then offered
> ego strengthening, deepening, and metaphors for control through
> acknowledgment and enhancement of spontaneous trance behaviors
> and relaxation through progressive relaxation.
>
> (Kohen, Mahowald, and Rosen 1992, 235–236)

The trance was deepened with progressive relaxation suggestions. The analogy of the brain being a computer and reprogramming to remove the bad habit was discussed. Participants were given instruction to practice self-hypnosis at home. A second session was held during which the experience of the past week was discussed and another hypnotic session was held which was audiotaped for the child to practice at home on a daily basis, alternating the hypnosis with and without the audiotape. A third session was held during which the experience was reviewed, and another hypnosis session was held for reinforcement. The children practiced RMI (self-hypnosis) daily over the next several months. All four patients remained symptom-free without medication during a two- to four-year follow-up.

Hauri, Silber, and Boeve (2007) reported on the treatment of 36 patients with various parasomnias with the use of hypnosis. Eleven had sleepwalking, ten had nightmares, six had sleep terrors, four had "epic dreaming," two had sleep-related eating disorder, one had sleep-related groaning, one had sleep-related hallucinations, and one had severe sleeptalking. The subjects ranged in age from six to 71 years. The initial evaluation began in the lead author's office where the use of hypnosis was discussed. They then moved to the sleep center bedroom where the patient was asked to lie on a bed concentrating on a spot on the ceiling. Guided imagery was carried out including the suggestion "they imagined a cloud coming down from the sky, enveloping them, and the patient then gradually dissolving into the cloud and floating through the sky as part of the cloud." The patients were then asked to imagine themselves in a movie,

> depicting how they were experiencing a good, parasomnia-free night of sleep at home. That is, they would see themselves go to bed, close their eyes, enter first a light, then a deeper stage of sleep, then the REM, etc., throughout the night.
>
> (Hauri, Silber, and Boeve 2007, 370)

Suggestions were given that they were safe and no longer needed the parasomnias and if the parasomnias occurred they could tell themselves "that it is no longer necessary." In order to test the depth of their hypnosis they were asked to fold their hands at the end of the session with the suggestion that their hands were glued together and could not be separated. Eight of the patients could easily separate their hands, when challenged to do so, which indicated to the author that they had not been hypnotized. An audiotape had been made of the session and they were instructed to practice it once a day for at least two weeks. They were told to come in for a follow-up session in two weeks if they needed it. Twenty-one of the patients canceled the appointment. Questionnaires were sent to the patients at one month, 18 months, and five-year follow-up. Overall, of those who returned the questionnaire, 42.2% were greatly improved after 18 months and 40.5% after five years. Of the six patients with sleepwalking who returned the questionnaire at 18 months, three were free from sleepwalking or much improved, as were two of three who returned the questionnaire after five years.

These cases demonstrate the successful use of hypnosis in treating sleepwalking utilizing various induction and post-hypnotic suggestion techniques. Hypnosis should be considered a treatment of choice for sleepwalking. It is self-empowering, inexpensive, safe, and the therapeutic effect is potentially long-lasting. Summarizing results from cases treated in his own Florida Sleep Institute, Dr. Kohler presented and described the following poster at the 4th International Congress of the World Association of Sleep Medicine (WASM), held in Quebec City, Canada, from September 10 through 14, 2011:

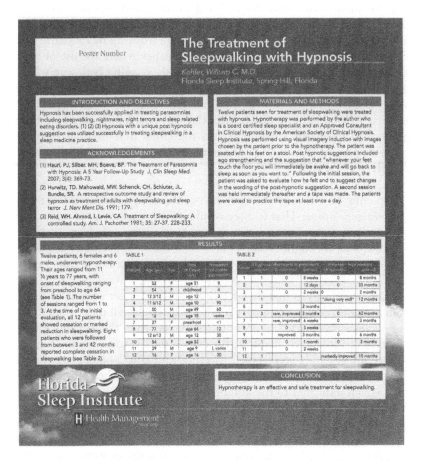

Figure 7.1 Hypnosis in the Treatment of Sleepwalking. Summary of a research
project conducted by William C. Kohler, M.D., at the Florida
Sleep Institute, Spring Hill, Florida, and presented in Quebec City
at WASM (2011). It was reproduced in Volume 12, September
2011 (Abstracts, Supplement 1, S1-S138), of *Sleep Medicine*, the
official journal of WASM and of the International Pediatric Sleep
Association, www.sleep-journal.com. A verbatim reproduction of the
contents of this poster is included in this work as Appendix B.)

Parasomnia Overlap Disorder

Parasomnia overlap disorder (POD) is a sleep disorder characterized by
the association of REM sleep parasomnia with an NREM sleep parasomnia in the same patient. RBD occurs in REM sleep with loss of inhibition
of motor pathways. The detailed underlying pathology is unclear. NREM
parasomnias, including sleepwalking, typically occur during slow-wave
sleep. There appears to be a genetic basis for both, but no definite gene

loci have been identified. Various central nervous system pathologies as well as medications have been associated with RBD, as summarized by Schenck and Howell (2013).

A review of the medical literature revealed relatively few cases of POD. Prior to 1997, only seven cases of potential POD were reported (Bokey 1993; Blanco and Garay 1995; Kushida et al. 1995). In 2013 Schenck and Howell reclassified POD, with the number of confirmed cases at that point up to 139.

Schenck, Boyd, and Mahowald (1997) reported 33 cases of POD involving sleepwalking, sleep terrors, and RBD confirmed by PSG. The report was based on a review and evaluation of 33 cases which were diagnosed at a clinical center during an eight-year period (1988–1996); these cases comprised approximately 21% of all RBD cases and 28% of all sleepwalking/ sleep terror cases seen at the center during that time period. Patients underwent clinical and PSG evaluations. The clinical evaluations included patient interviews and the completion of a structured questionnaire. Mean age of parasomnia onset ranged from one to 60 years; 70% ($n = 23$) were males. According to the summary, "Forty-five percent ($n = 15$) had previously received psychological or psychiatric therapy for their parasomnia without benefit." Treatment outcome "was available for $n = 20$ patients; 90% ($n = 18$) had substantial parasomnia control with bedtime clonazepam ($n = 13$), alprazolam and/or carbamazepine ($n = 4$), or self hypnosis ($n = 1$)." However there were no details concerning the case treated with hypnosis. The summary concluded that "parasomnia overlap disorder is a treatable condition that emerges in various clinical settings and can be understood within the context of current knowledge on parasomnias and motor control/dyscontrol during sleep" (Schenck, Boyd, and Mahowald 1997, 972).

Alves et al. (1999) published a case of a 27-year-old with sexual behavior during sleep (SBS) which they felt was a case of probable parasomnia overlap syndrome. He had a history of sleepwalking since age nine and developed disruptive violent nocturnal behavior with dream enactment at age 20 with injurious behavior to himself, his wife, and infant. He was also amnestic to sexual activity occurring during sleep. Remarkable clinical improvement was noted using clonazepam 2 mg at bedtime.

Bonakis et al. (2009) retrospectively evaluated 91 patients with RBD. They were divided into two groups: over age 50 and under age 50. The <50 group consisted of 23 male and 16 female patients. Twenty had idiopathic RBD and 19 secondary RBD. Among the patients with idiopathic RBD, 13 had complex behavior, including episodes of sleeptalking and sleepwalking. In the group of patients older than 50, there were 39 males and 13 females. Thirty-three had a diagnosis of idiopathic RBD, of whom two also experienced behavior compatible with sleepwalking. The researchers concluded that there was a very strong association between RBD and NREM parasomnias. They found that this was not uncommon in cases of idiopathic RBD affecting patients below age 50. The presence of a REM parasomnia (in this case RBD) and an NREM parasomnia forms the diagnosis of POD.

Limousin et al. (2009) reported on a case of a brainstem inflammatory lesion in the pontine tegmentum causing RBD and sleepwalking. They hypothesized that a unilateral lesion by itself was sufficient to cause both the RBD and sleepwalking. They suggested that unilateral lesions of the REM sleep atonia system are sufficient to enhance/release axial and bilateral limb muscle tone during REM sleep and also to trigger sleepwalking. Melatonin, 9 mg per day, improved the symptoms but clonazepam did not.

Cicolin et al. (2011) reported 2 patients with SBS associated with POD documented by PSG, with video-PSG documentation of sexual behavior in one of the two cases. One patient was a 60-year-old female in whom SBS was demonstrated on video-PSG. An episode of masturbation occurring during slow-wave sleep and preceded by hypersynchronous delta pattern was recorded. The EEG pattern showed the persistence of delta rhythms with increasing alpha activity. According to the abstract, "when awoken by technicians, the patient was not aware of her sexual behavior and did not report any dreams." She had a history of sleeptalking and sleepwalking since childhood. There was also a four-year history of motor activity occurring in the second half of the night, often violent, and associated with vivid dreams.

The episodes with the second patient, a 41-year-old male, documented a case of POD by PSG. He had a history of engaging in sexual behavior (fondling and/or intercourse) while asleep. There was a history of sleepwalking since childhood and over the past six years he had developed episodes of violent behavior, occasionally self-injurious, with dream content. According to the abstract, "this is an unprecedented report of SBS in patients with PSG-confirmed POD and of SBS documented during video-PSG" (Cicolin et al. 2011, 523).

Dumitrascu et al. (2013) reported five individuals with POD where the arousal, non-REM parasomnia, was the more prominent feature than the RBD component. After analyzing their cases and those reported in the literature they concluded that POD is most likely a separate condition and not a subtype of RBD. The *International Classification of Sleep Disorders* (2nd edition; American Academy of Sleep Medicine 2005), identifies POD as a variant of RBD rather than a separate disorder.

A review of the literature revealed no detailed cases of POD treated with hypnosis other than the case reported by the authors in 2014 (Kohler, Kurz, and Kohler 2014). This case is reviewed in detail in Chapter 9.

Nightmares

Nightmares are a parasomnia occurring during REM sleep. Dreams are frightening and usually involve anxiety, but anger, rage, or other negative feelings may occur. Nightmares are common; up to 90% of people complain of having at least occasional nightmares. As opposed to night terrors, nightmares are more common and are usually remembered, at times with great detail. Trauma-related nightmares are common in patients with post-traumatic stress disorder (PTSD). Certain medications and food are known to elicit nightmares, as does alcohol and drug withdrawal. There appears to be a genetic influence.

Most cases of nightmares are benign and need no treatment. However, at times they are severe enough to interfere with daytime functioning. Numerous treatments have been reported, including imagery rehearsal, psychotherapy, relaxation techniques, lucid dreaming, and hypnosis.

Linden, Bhardwaj, and Anbar (2006) reported on the use of hypnosis to treat nightmares in 11 children and adolescents ranging in age from 11 to 20 years. Three induction techniques were taught:

> (1) their hands were giant magnets that attracted one another, and noticing how the hands came together, "on their own," (2) that they were holding a bucket full of heavy wet sand in one raised hand and noticing how it became heavy, and (3) that they were holding a handful of helium balloons of various colors, and noticing how their hand became lighter intended to rise, "all by itself."
>
> (Linden, Bhardwaj, and Anbar 2006, 283)

Relaxation imagery was utilized and individuals were taught how to use a gesture to remind them how to relax. Instruction in the induction and relaxation techniques took approximately 15 minutes. In the first or second hypnotic session one of two methods was used to hypnotically induce dream recall in order to help process their dreams. If the patient was frightened by the dream content they:

> were offered an opportunity to review the dreams within a 10 cm diameter crystal ball after they achieved a state of hypnosis by imagining their relaxing place. It was suggested that the dream would not be as frightening because it would be seen in the crystal ball rather than inside the child's mind.

A second method was the suggestion "that once they were in a relaxed state with the aid of hypnosis, they would begin to dream their nightmare." Under hypnosis, when their nightmare reached the point when they would usually awaken they were encouraged to continue in hypnosis and allow the dream to reach its conclusion. They were asked to define the meaning of the dream. In all the patients, the nightmares were reported to have decreased in frequency or completely resolved (Linden, Bhardwaj, and Anbar 2006, 383–384).

Hauri, Silber, and Boeve (2007), as discussed in the section on sleepwalking (somnambulism), reported on the use of hypnosis in 36 patients with various parasomnias. Ten of the patients had nightmares. Questionnaires revealed that after 18 months five of seven patients were free from nightmares or much improved and after five years four of six were nightmare-free.

Hypnosis can be a very effective tool in reducing or completely eliminating nightmares.

Nocturnal Enuresis

Nocturnal enuresis (sleep enuresis, bedwetting) is the involuntary act of urinating at night. It is very common and affects millions of children and some adults. There are basically two types of enuresis. In primary enuresis the child has never been consistently dry at night. Developmentally the child's brain has not learned to awaken at a signal from the bladder that it is full. In secondary enuresis the child has been consistently dry for at least six months and begins bedwetting again. This may be triggered by stress or be the result of an underlying urinary tract infection, diabetes, or other medical condition, including sleep disorders such as obstructive sleep apnea.

Children develop control over their bladder at different ages and there appears to be a genetic component. It is considered abnormal if the child is still wetting the bed more than twice a month after age five or six. Some clinicians do not consider bedwetting to be abnormal unless it occurs more than twice a month after six years of age for girls or seven years of age for boys. Most children achieve bladder control by four years of age. It is estimated that, at age five, 16% of children are still having nocturnal enuresis, 13% at age six and 1–2% are still wetting the bed at age 15. Bedwetting is more common in boys.

If primary nocturnal enuresis persists longer than age six or seven, and if it is causing significant social problems or secondary enuresis develops, an evaluation by a physician is indicated. A complete history and physical should be obtained along with urinalysis. If an underlying cause is found, treatment should be specific for that condition. However, only in a small minority of patients will a specific etiology be ascertained. Treatment for most cases of nocturnal enuresis requires nothing more than reassurance that bedwetting is common, that almost all children will outgrow it, and that it can be treated. Limiting fluid intake close to bedtime and avoiding punishment or embarrassing the child are appropriate early steps. Waterproof mattress pads and absorbent underwear may be indicated. Bedwetting alarms which sound a loud tone when they sense moisture have been found to be effective in some patients. Medication such as DDAVP (desmopressin) reduces urine production during sleep. Tricyclic antidepressants such as imipramine, amitriptyline, and nortriptyline reduce the rate of enuresis but, like DDAVP, can have potentially dangerous side-effects. Anticipatory wakening may be beneficial if the child routinely has a bedwetting episode at the same time each night and is awakened prior to the episode. Sphincter control exercises, bladder expansion (drinking excessive fluid during the day and holding back the urine as long as you can), and star charts (placing a star on a chart each time the child is dry) have also been utilized.

Hypnosis is a technique that can significantly improve nocturnal enuresis without the side-effects of medication. It has been used for many years to treat nocturnal enuresis and there are numerous published accounts indicating the efficacy of hypnotherapy in treating nocturnal enuresis. A brief review of several of these reports is summarized below.

Collison (1970) reported on the use of hypnosis to treat 11 patients with secondary enuresis (also called onset nocturnal enuresis). Ages ranged from 5½ to 38 years and included nine males and two females. All had been treated previously with other methods for enuresis without success. Once the patients were in a trance direct suggestions were made that they would be dry at night, and given suggestions for ego strengthening and social adjustment. The therapist also utilized age regression and abreaction to uncover any potential dramatic events that led to the enuresis. Each of the patients reportedly had a specific precipitating stress or were members of families that had high levels of tension at the time of the onset of enuresis. The suggestion was also given that if the bladder required emptying during the night the patient would awaken and use the toilet before the bed became wet. Each session lasted from 15 minutes to one hour and was repeated for six to 20 weeks. Nine of the patients were "dry" at follow-up between three and five years. Two of the patients remained "wet" on follow-up at one year and 4½ years.

Olness (1975) described the treatment with hypnosis of 40 children ranging in age from four to 16 years. Twenty had primary nocturnal enuresis and 20 had "onset" nocturnal enuresis. The two teenagers in the group were taught the "hand levitation" induction technique whereas the 38 younger patients were taught the "coin" technique. The initial interview took 10–25 minutes and each follow-up took 5–10 minutes. Direct suggestions were made that the children were to review daily. At the time of the report the children had been followed from 6 to 28 months. In 31 of the children the bedwetting had resolved, in six there was a decrease in frequency of enuresis, whereas three did not improve. The children who were successful required no more than two visits before improvement was noted.

Edwards and van der Spuy (1985) reported on the treatment of 48 boys, ages 8–13 – 24 with primary nocturnal enuresis and 24 with secondary enuresis – who were randomly assigned to four different treatment protocols. Six with primary enuresis and six with secondary enuresis were assigned to each protocol. In Protocol One, trance was induced with the suggestion of relaxation and that the patients were entering a unique state. These suggestions were made by tape through headphones. Post-hypnotic suggestions of tension reduction and enhancement of self-confidence were made. Suggestions for increased bladder capacity, fluid reduction before bedtime, urinating before bedtime, and awakening at night to urinate on experiencing a full bladder were made. In Protocol Two the same suggestions were made as in Protocol One but there was no induction of a trance first. In Protocol Three, prior to induction patients were advised that hypnosis would help them become dry and more confident and independent. Then trance was induced and they were awakened from the trance without further suggestions after a few minutes. In Protocol Four, no treatment was performed initially. Patients were offered treatment at the six-month follow-up. Six weekly one-hour sessions were held over a six-week period. The researchers reported that at the six-month evaluation hypnotherapy was significantly effective in decreasing nocturnal enuresis compared to the pretreatment baseline enuresis frequency and to the no-treatment condition. They also found that trance induction was not necessary for success.

Bannerjee, Srivastav, and Palan (1993) compared treatment with hypnotherapy to imipramine in two groups, each group consisting of 25 children with enuresis ranging in age from five to 16. Forty-four children had primary enuresis and six had secondary enuresis. The physiology and anatomy of urinary control were explained to the children in the hypnosis treatment group by utilizing simple line diagrams. Explanations were given that their brain gave signals to all parts of the body for it to appropriately function and that they were going to learn a technique to have their brain control the urinary bladder. Hypnosis was induced utilizing visual imagery. Suggestions were given that they would awaken from a dry bed when the bladder was full, walk to the bathroom, urinate in the toilet, return to a dry bed, and go back to sleep. During the first week two 30-minute sessions were held with one additional session being held the next week. The children were advised to use self-hypnosis every night prior to going to bed. Subsequent sessions were held depending on the response of the child. The children in the imipramine group were initially treated with 25 mg every night. The dose was increased every seven days depending upon the response. Follow-up visits occurred weekly for the first month and then monthly for two additional months. At the three-month visit the imipramine was discontinued. The children in the hypnosis group were advised to practice self-hypnosis nightly. Seventy-two percent of the hypnosis group and 76% of the imipramine group were reported to have a positive treatment outcome at the three-month evaluation. At nine months, 68% of the hypnosis group were reported to have a positive result compared to 24% of the imipramine group (who had been without treatment for the past six months).

In spite of the many reports of the successful use of hypnosis in the treatment of nocturnal enuresis there has been a lack of classical controlled studies showing its efficacy. As discussed previously, based on the nature of hypnosis, controlled studies are very difficult to accomplish. Nevertheless, the studies that are available demonstrate that hypnosis is a valuable technique for treating nocturnal enuresis.

Bruxism

Bruxism is grinding or clenching of the teeth. It may occur during wakefulness or during sleep. Bruxism may occur at any age. It has been reported that 85–90% of the population will have bruxism at some point during their life. Sleep bruxism, even in chronic bruxers, may skip several nights only to return. There is no clear cause for bruxism but it has been associated with stress and emotional tension. Bruxism causes an unpleasant noise which may disrupt the sleep of the bruxer and/or bed partner. Bruxism may lead to abnormal tooth wear, myofascial pain, headaches, and temporomandibular joint dysfunction. It can be recognized during an overnight PSG by increased masseter and temporalis muscle activity and is most common in stage N2 sleep but can occur in all stages.

Numerous therapies have been utilized to control bruxism, including relaxation and biofeedback training, medication, dental splints, and psychotherapy, as well as hypnosis. As with other uses of hypnosis, it is not a stand-alone technique but is used in conjunction with other therapies. Underlying medical or dental causes for bruxism should be ruled out before treatment with hypnosis is started.

Clarke and Reynolds (1991) reported on the use of hypnosis in eight subjects with bruxism. They termed their treatment approach "suggestive hypnotherapy." In Session One a number of hypnotic images, deepening techniques, and inductions were suggested. The phrase "lips together, teeth apart" was suggested, as were images such as hot towels on the face. Patient preferences were utilized in Session Two, when an audiotape was made that was to be practiced each night. The tape was 8–10 minutes long and ended with "sleep suggestions." A third session was held including a short hypnosis session. A total of four to eight sessions were held over 2–4 months. Posttreatment electromyogram activity of bruxism was measured and was significantly lower than pretreatment recordings, which correlated with the self-reports of improvement.

Somer (1991) reported on a case of bruxism successfully treated with hypnosis. He postulated that the treatment needed to be twofold – the potential cause of conflict fueling the muscle tension needed to be identified and then the muscle tension needed to be controlled. His patient was a 55-year-old male with a long history of nocturnal and diurnal bruxism. There was no underlying anatomical cause for the bruxism. He had been prescribed a dental splint. Several sessions were held exploring childhood experiences that could possibly be associated with his current tension. A hypnosis session was held with eye fixation (where the patient is asked to look at a point or an object) and body relaxation induction (suggestions for relaxation of muscle groups; in the case of bruxism the suggestion was for relaxation of jaw muscles). Trance was deepened and a hypnoanalytic exploration (hypnosis integrated with psychoanalytic techniques) was conducted, revealing that conflict with his father had been reactivated in his current work environment. At the time of the seventh session cognitive behavioral hypnosis was conducted with the suggestion that his mouth would be more relaxed during sleep and he would awaken if he attempted to grind his teeth. The 20-minute session was audiotaped and he was asked to play it every night prior to bedtime. Telephone follow-up at 3 and 12 months found the patient to be sleeping well without the dental splint and with no significant discomfort.

Dowd (2013) discussed possible causes and treatment of bruxism in a review of the literature and presented a case of bruxism that was successfully treated with hypnotherapy. Hypnotic intervention focused mainly on the psychological aspects of the bruxism, not the muscular aspect of it. The patient was a 33-year-old female who had a history of bruxism dating back many years. Severe bruxism at night was present. She wore mouth guards but would wear them out in 6 months or less. There was no evidence of a medical or dental problem causing the bruxism. Potential causes of stress were explored. During the second session a hypnotic routine was carried out with suggestions that "her unconscious mind would begin to learn new ways of acting in the world." At the time of the third session significant improvement was reported. Another hypnotic routine was conducted "around themes of shedding old roles in life and old discomfort and pain." During the fourth session another hypnotherapy induction was carried out with "themes of making new connections among her thoughts, feelings, and actions as she grows and develops." Three more sessions were carried out. A phone call follow-up a year later revealed that her jaw pain had not returned and that her relationships with her family had improved (Dowd 2013, 211–212).

These cases point out different hypnotherapeutic approaches with different induction techniques and different post-hypnotic suggestions. They also emphasize a complete evaluation of the patient prior to employing hypnosis. These are case reports rather than controlled studies but do point out the utility of hypnosis in correcting bruxism. As mentioned previously, hypnosis does not yield itself readily to controlled trials since the interaction between the hypnotherapist and the patient is crucial and does not lend itself readily to a static script.

Night Terrors

Night terrors (*pavor nocturnus*) are a disorder of arousal typically occurring in NREM slow-wave sleep; sleepwalking also occurs during NREM slow-wave sleep. The behavior often occurs during the transition between deep and light sleep in what is considered a "partial arousal." This arousal response can be triggered by external stimuli. An important difference between sleepwalking and night terror is that in the former there is no fear. Piercing screams or incoherent vocalizations and behaviors consistent with intense fear – along with signs of intense autonomic activity – occur in night terrors. Flushing of the skin, sweating, tachycardia, increased muscle tone, and pupil dilatation may be present. Occasionally the patient bolts out of bed and runs. Violent behavior can occur. Confusion and disorientation may be present. The patient is amnestic for the episodes although occasional reports of fragmentary dreaming may occur. Night terrors may occur at any age. Up to 6.5% of children and 2.2% of adults are reported to experience night terrors. As noted in the discussion of sleepwalking, genetics may play a role in this NREM parasomnia. Other sleep disorders such as obstructive sleep apnea, psychiatric disorders, and anxiety may also play a role. Sleep deprivation, emotional stress, medications, and alcohol can cause sleep terrors. Typically in children there is no underlying psychopathology. In children, night terrors, like sleepwalking, tend to resolve spontaneously during adolescence. As with any medical condition, before treatment is begun a thorough evaluation should be carried out in an attempt to find the underlying cause. Psychotherapy has been helpful in cases where the cause is associated with psychological trauma and stress. Medications such as antidepressants and tranquilizers have been noted to have efficacy. Hypnosis has also been found to be an effective form of treatment, as noted by the cases below.

Koe (1989) reported the successful use of hypnosis in a 16-year-old male for whom other forms of treatment for night terrors had failed. He had night terrors dating back to age seven. The episodes consisted of repetitive screaming and leaping out of bed and running around the room. At times he became violent during the episodes. During the agitated aspect of his night terror he broke his mother's nose, smashed a window, and threw objects around the room. He had been treated with psychotherapy and tranquilizers without success. The Harvard Group Scale of Hypnotic Susceptibility was used to evaluate his possible response to hypnosis and the Long Stanford Scale of Hypnotic Depth was used to indicate the depth of hypnosis. A systematic relaxation induction was utilized. Suggestions were given that he was in deep sleep, the stage where he usually experienced night terrors, and that a night terror was beginning. His respiratory rate was noted to accelerate. Autonomic activity increased and the therapist tapped his desk lightly with a pencil, at which point the patient began screaming, jumped up, and ran into a wall. He was confused and disoriented. A week later he was again hypnotized and was given the post-hypnotic suggestion that he would become less and less aware of outside noises and sensations while asleep. This suggestion was repeated several times. At follow-up evaluation in three months it was reported that his night terrors had resolved. The therapist suggested that the arousal phenomena was from external noise and that the post-hypnotic suggestion to reduce the awareness of this contributed to the success of the hypnosis.

Kramer (1989) described the use of hypnosis in a ten-year-old male who had experienced night terrors since age four. The episodes occurred approximately four times per week and started 20 minutes after sleep onset. Hypnotic induction was carried out by the finger-lowering technique where he was asked to raise the middle two fingers and then watch them as they "go to sleep." While in trance the nature of sleep was explained stage by stage with emphasis on the continual movement of sleep cycles. "He was also given direct suggestions for not dropping too quickly into an extremely deep stage of sleep." A second session was held a week later and the above suggestions were reinforced. A follow-up approximately two years later revealed that he continued to be free from night terrors (Kramer 1989, 284).

Hurwitz et al. (1991), as discussed in the section on sleepwalking, utilized hypnosis to treat 27 adults with sleepwalking and sleep terrors. Four of the patients had sleep terrors and 15 had a combination of sleep terrors and sleepwalking. Seventy-four percent of the 27 patients reported having significant improvement when contacted between 6 and 63 months after treatment.

Kohen, Mahowald, and Rosen (1992), as noted above in the discussion of the use of hypnosis in sleepwalking, successfully treated with hypnotherapy four children who had NREM parasomnias. Two of the children had sleep terrors in addition to sleepwalking. All the children were reported to be symptom-free during a 2–4-year follow-up without having to utilize medication.

Hoogduin and Hagenaars (2000) reported on the use of hypnosis in treating four patients with night terrors. Treatment consisted of initial gathering of information concerning the night terrors from memory fragments the patient may have had and from reports of other observers such as family members. The hypnotic trance was induced utilizing "fixation." While in the trance two patients were allowed to relive threatening situations that had been previously gathered. It was suggested that there was nothing to fear. Suggestions for relaxation and stress reduction were made. An audiotape was made which they were to practice prior to going to sleep each night or several times per day. Follow-up sessions were held. The duration of therapy varied. All patients were considered to have positive results with improvement of night terrors from 50% to 100%.

Hauri, Silber, and Boeve (2007), as noted in the discussion of the use of hypnosis in sleepwalking, reported on the use of hypnosis in 36 patients ranging in age from six to 71. Six of the patients had sleep terrors. At follow-up in 18 months, one out of five reported being free of sleep terrors or much improved, with one in four reporting this after five years.

These cases demonstrate various rates of success and utilized different hypnotic techniques. All of the cases demonstrated that hypnosis was safe and in many cases improved or eliminated the night terrors.

Sleep Paralysis

Sleep paralysis is a parasomnia occurring during REM sleep. There is inability to perform voluntary movement, speak, or even move the fingers. The paralysis appears to be similar to the change in muscle tone that occurs in normal REM sleep, where alpha motor neurones are hyperpolarized. The episodes may occur at sleep onset (hypnagogic), or upon awakening during the night or in the morning (hypnopompic). Sleep paralysis may occur as an isolated event, most commonly on awakening, or in narcolepsy where it may be more prevalent at sleep onset. It may also occur in a familial form and may be transmitted as an X-linked dominant trait. Hypnagogic hallucinations, auditory and tactile, may accompany sleep paralysis, making the episodes even more frightening. Predisposing factors may include sleep deprivation, irregular sleep habits, sleeping in the supine position, and mental stress. The episodes usually last minutes but can rarely extend to hours. The events are spontaneously terminated or terminate after the patient is touched or alerted to a sound. Isolated sleep paralysis is common and needs no intervention other than reassurance that the episodes are benign. However, when the episodes are frequent and interfere with the patient's sleep, cause severe anxiety, or interfere with daytime functioning then therapeutic intervention is indicated.

Nardi (1981) reported two cases of sleep paralysis which were successfully treated with hypnosis. The first case was a 25-year-old female who had separated from her husband of four years. She reported that her first recent attack had taken place shortly after her marriage, but had a vague memory of two episodes when she was much younger. The sleep paralysis caused extreme fright. She related to Dr. Nardi that she thought she was "stuck in this body and people are going to think I'm dead." She remained awake the rest of the night for fear of another attack. The attacks occurred approximately once per month, but apparently did not continue to be frightening experiences. She was taught self-hypnosis as a way of being more in control. The initial hypnotic induction was "by progressive relaxation and then deepened by arm levitation." (In arm levitation patients are advised to concentrate on the sensations in their fingers and hand, and the hand will tend to lift itself and float towards the face.) She was told that even though she was "very relaxed and motionless her mind could still control her body and direct her arm to rise." She was advised to "enjoy the relaxed motionless state that she could end whenever she wanted." She was brought out of the trance by a count from five to one and was instructed to take three deep slow breaths and relax as deeply as she had been. She was advised to enjoy the relaxation and then count herself out of it. The procedure was repeated again and then the session was terminated. She was to practice the technique twice a day. She was advised that when the next episode of sleep paralysis occurred she was not to force herself to awaken but to take three deep breaths and purposely relax. She was then to decide whether to relax and enjoy the experience, fall back to sleep, or awaken herself by counting herself out of the self-hypnosis, and hence out of the sleep paralysis. At the next session she was assisted in learning how to deepen the self-hypnosis. She was followed for more than 14 months and was successful in either relaxing enough to fall back to sleep when the attacks of sleep paralysis occurred or to completely awaken (Nardi 1981, 360–361).

The second case was a 30-year-old female who had requested hypnosis for her fear of flying. She was taught self-hypnosis using the same technique as in the previous case. She was also given suggestions concerning relaxation and enjoyment of the flight. Several sessions were held before her flight for reinforcement and deepening of the trance. When she returned following the travel, she reported that she had a good experience except for a strange episode where she awoke in her hotel room unable to move or scream and saw a man standing motionless in the room. In retrospect she described episodes of sleep paralysis dating back to age six. The episodes occurred five to six times per year and were always frightening but she never had had a visual hallucination previously. She was instructed to utilize self-hypnosis when the next attack occurred. She was further instructed to decide if she wanted to relax and go back to sleep or count herself out of the episode and hence out of the sleep paralysis. She was told that the appearance of someone in her room was actually part of a dream state that at times accompanies sleep paralysis. She was instructed that the dream would vanish when she came out of the self-hypnosis. Over the next ten months two or three episodes occurred which she was able to handle successfully. She also had a few hypnagogic hallucinations that were non-threatening.

Hallucinations

Hallucinations are vivid dreamlike perceptions that may occur at sleep onset (hypnagogic) or while awakening during the night (hypnopompic). These hallucinations may be part of a normal sleep phenomenon or may be terrifying and result in insomnia and daytime sequelae. Hallucinations may involve visual, auditory, or tactile phenomena. Gustatory and proprioceptive hallucinations may also occur. Hallucinations are normal phenomena but can be part of underlying psychiatric illness. They may be caused by medications or neurodegenerative processes or be associated with narcolepsy.

Ortega (1984) reported on a case of severe frightening hypnopompic hallucinations treated by hypnotic techniques. The patient was a 21-year-old male who, on awakening, perceived creatures in the bedroom that were humanlike and of which he was terrified. He threw objects, including books and clocks, at the images. This was dangerous for anyone in the room at the time of the hallucinations. It took half an hour to an hour for him to regain his composure before he could start the day. The hallucinations dated back 12 years and occurred approximately every ten days. A hypnotic trance was induced utilizing the arm levitation technique as well as the escalator deepening technique. Direct suggestions were made for the patient not to observe the hallucinatory images "but to focus on watching himself remain calm during a frightening hallucination." These instructions were made for the first four sessions. During the next sessions he was instructed to actually have his hypnopompic hallucinations "in their full intensity moving about the room while he remained calm and relaxed." Direct suggestions that the patient would no longer have hypnopompic hallucinations were made during the final two weeks of therapy. At the patient's six-month follow-up it was reported that he had not had any "transitional state hallucinations" (Ortega 1984, 112).

Treatment options for idiopathic hypnopompic hallucinations are limited. Hypnosis offers a possible viable therapy for this condition.

CPAP Compliance

Obstructive sleep apnea is a significant cause of mortality and morbidity. It affects the quality of life as well as contributes to significant medical problems. Hypertension, excessive daytime somnolence, impaired cognition, depression, cardiovascular disease, cerebrovascular disease, increased risk of accidents, impotence in males, and abnormalities in glucose and cholesterol metabolism have been associated with obstructive sleep apnea. In children, failure to thrive, cor pulmonale (failure of the right side of the heart), developmental delay, impaired cognition, and behavioral dysfunction have been attributed to obstructive sleep apnea.

There is no satisfactory way to diagnose apnea without doing a PSG. However, if you snore, are tired during the day, or have a neck circumference of 17 inches in males or 15 inches in females, sleep apnea should be considered.

Since apnea contributes to significant medical problems such as those noted above, it is important to treat the apnea effectively.

Up to the present time, the most effective therapy for obstructive sleep apnea is continuous positive airway pressure (CPAP). The main obstacle to successful therapy is non-compliance with CPAP use. Various studies have shown up to 50% of obstructive sleep apnea patients prescribed CPAP are poorly compliant. One of the most important factors to CPAP compliance is the comfort of the CPAP mask. This has resulted in the development of hundreds of different styles of masks. Interventions such as medication, humidification, alternative pressure delivery systems such as autoPAP and flexible bilevel airway pressure, in addition to education programs have been attempted with mixed results.

Sometimes people worry about feeling claustrophobic, looking "funny," or having trouble learning to use the equipment with its buttons and cleaning requirements.

Reducing anxiety and stress by utilizing the CPAP mask while watching TV to become more comfortable with it sometimes helps. Suggestions for patients to prop up their feet and watch a favorite movie while utilizing CPAP may be given. Behavioral approaches such as cognitive behavioral therapy may also be of help.

Hypnosis has a potentially important role in CPAP compliance but has infrequently been utilized; there are very few published reports concerning its efficacy.

Khirani et al. (2013) reported a case where hypnosis was utilized to facilitate CPAP acceptance in a child with cherubism who had severe obstructive sleep apnea. (Cherubism is a rare genetic disorder with the abnormal growth of giant cell lesions of the lower jaw producing a cherub-like facial appearance.) A PSG revealed "profound desaturations and the need for a CPAP therapy." Treatment was complicated because of high anticipatory anxiety and complete choanal obstruction rendering the use of a nasal mask impossible. An oral mask interface was utilized. Hypnosis was administered by a trained nurse. Details of the procedure were not presented. The report indicated that "different consecutive hypnotic induction techniques were successfully used." The patient reportedly accepted CPAP after three sessions of hypnosis. It was reported that compliance with CPAP was about eight hours after one week of use (Khirani et al. 2013, 928–929).

DeLord et al. (2013) reported on the use of hypnosis in nine children ranging in age from two to 15 to acclimatize them to the successful use of non-invasive positive-pressure ventilation (NPPV). This is the same group of authors that reported the case noted above. The hypnosis was administered by a nurse trained in hypnotic technique. Depending on the age of the child, various hypnotic techniques were utilized. In the two-year-old patient distraction with visual, auditory, and kinesthetic stimulation was carried out. In older children either indirect suggestions were utilized, with children expressing their imagination spontaneously and the therapist accompanying children in the imaginary experience or direct suggestions where the therapist gave direct suggestions to help them enter the imaginary experience. The individual sessions lasted 15–30 minutes and were repeated later that day or the next day at the child's request. Parents were free to attend the sessions. Success was measured by the acceptance of NPPV by the patient. All patients accepted NPPV at the first daytime session. However, for overnight acceptance it took a median of three sessions. Long-term compliance was measured by a memory chip in the home ventilators. There was a median objective compliance of 7.5 hours per night in eight of the nine patients at six months. A 15-year-old patient with severe obstructive sleep apnea and morbid obesity underwent bariatric surgery so long-term therapy with NPPV was not necessary.

In these cases the anticipatory anxiety concerning the procedure was reduced or eliminated. This approach is applicable for both children and adults. When anxiety is present, hypnosis has a particularly powerful role in relieving that anxiety. Sleep clinicians and their patients need to be aware of this valuable tool for improving CPAP compliance.

Post-Traumatic Stress Disorder (PTSD)

Diagnostic criteria published in *Diagnosis and Statistical Manual of Mental Disorders*, fourth and fifth edition (DSM-IV and DSM-V: American Psychiatric Association, 2000, 2013) and *International Classification of Diseases*, ninth and 10th editions (ICD-9 and ICD-10: World Health Organization, 1979, 2015) vary. PTSD symptoms can develop following any serious psychological trauma. Experiencing or witnessing a severe event or threat to oneself or others where a sensation of powerlessness, horror, and fear are felt can result in PTSD. The reaction to severe stress depends on the individual's underlying genetics, as well as previous experience and coping mechanisms. Upsetting memories and the replaying of images in one's mind, not the direct experience of the traumatic event itself, perpetuates the symptoms of PTSD. Images take on a life of their own.

The term PTSD was first coined in the 1970s. Over the years the criteria for diagnosing PTSD have changed. Diagnostic criteria published in *Diagnostic and Statistical Manual of Mental Disorders*, 4th edn (DSM-IV) and DSM-V and *International Classification of Diseases*, 9th revision (ICD-9) and ICD-10 vary. Previously, similar symptoms were referred to in terms such as anxiety or war neuroses.

There are various pharmacologic and psychological interventions to improve symptoms of PTSD or to attempt to prevent them from occurring after a traumatic experience.

As an intervention technique, hypnosis allows the person to experience the image more vividly and assist in assimilation. The use of imagery has been beneficial for induction of the hypnotic state, for deepening of that state, and for changing behavior. Hypnotic techniques can be used to alter and assimilate the traumatic experience and the recurring images.

Watkins utilized hypnosis in successfully treating traumatic war neuroses at the Army's Welch Convalescent Hospital in Daytona Beach, Florida, in the 1940s. This is one of the early reports of the successful use of hypnosis in a large number of patients for a condition that later became known as PTSD (Watkins 1987).

Appel (1999) described the use of hypnosis in reframing intrusive imagery. Significant distress is created as the mind replays the traumatic experiences. Changing the image allows the mind to assimilate it in a form that reduces or eliminates this distress. Appel presented four cases with different types of intrusive imagery that were successfully treated with hypnosis, three of which will briefly discussed.

Case One

A 35-year-old female had sustained multiple musculoskeletal injuries in a car accident. A year and a half later she witnessed the traumatic amputation of a leg in a motorcycle crash. She then assisted providing first aid. She developed intrusive images of the driver and the severed leg. Under hypnosis she was asked to place the intrusive image on a TV set and as she moved back from the set she would note that she was looking at one of several television sets. As she continued moving back there would be more TV sets showing different scenes from her life. As she moved back more television sets were present and she could choose to pay attention to any particular TV or numbers of sets that she chose. It was suggested that:

> just as it was difficult for her to focus on the particular TV with the accident amongst all the other TVs from that distance, any time she needed to have perspective, she could put the memory of the accident in its proper perspective as she had just done.

This single intervention ameliorated her symptoms.

Case Two

A nine-year-old girl had repeated nightmares of a fiendish murderer who wore a bag over his head. Under hypnosis she was asked to visualize a movie studio where she was to sit next to the director viewing the various stagehands, then watch the murderer "come out, trip and fall, and tear his paper bag." She was assisted in viewing the event several times in the making of one scene. "She was helped to consciously re-realize an existing schema related to movie production and the image was treated as a frame in a movie about making a movie." Her symptoms abated after this single intervention.

Case Three

A 60-year-old male had a childhood history of abuse with recurrent impulses to cry and scream and the impression that he was "hearing in his head his aunt and uncle accusing him of being a cry baby and other negative associations." Under hypnosis he was instructed to imagine himself as a young boy and place into a TV set the image of his aunt and uncle making the harmful statements. He was to visualize numerous TVs, as was done in Case Two, above. He was to visualize himself in positive roles in other TV sets next to the TV holding the uncomfortable memory. He was instructed to view all the images "and realize who he was and what his life was about." This technique was successful in reducing the intrusive images (Appel 1999, 331).

Lynn et al. (2012) reviewed the use of hypnosis in treating PTSD. Cognitive behavioral therapy was reviewed in conjunction with hypnosis. They suggested that hypnosis was "fundamentally a cognitive-behavioral intervention" and that "hypnosis can be a useful adjunct to evidence-based cognitive-behavioral approaches" in the treatment of PTSD (Lynn et al. 2012, 311).

Over a decade ago, a sleep specialist asked me (WCK) to evaluate a hospital chaplain who had also been a chaplain in the military and who was experiencing severe insomnia secondary to recurrent nightmares which were felt to be part of PTSD. I utilized my regular visual imagery induction. The post-hypnotic suggestions were that the images were vapors and could not cause harm to him. They did not harm him in the past and would not harm him now or in the future. This was repeated several times with suggestions for ego strengthening. An audiotape was made which he practiced. On follow-up a month later his symptoms had resolved.

Rhythmic Movement Disorder

Rhythmic movement disorder is a sleep–wake transition disorder parasomnia and refers to a group of repetitive movements typically occurring prior to sleep onset which may continue on into light sleep. The most common form is head banging. Head rolling, body rocking, body rolling, leg banging, and leg rolling may also occur. Rhythmic movement disorder of some form occurs in most infants and usually dissipates by age four. It can occur in older children and adults and may be associated with psychopathology, autism, and mental retardation. Chanting or rhythmic humming may be present. It is more prevalent in males and may be familial. The rocking may have a soothing effect.

Headbanging (*jactatio capitis nocturna*) is the most common and potentially the most harmful rhythmic movement disorder. Head injury is uncommon but may occur. Retinal petechiae and subdural hematoma have been reported.

There have been no controlled studies showing an ideal treatment regimen. Pharmacologic and behavioral interventions have been reported. Protecting the bed environment to avoid head injury has been beneficial.

Several case studies have documented the successful use of hypnosis in rhythmic movement disorder.

Rosenberg (1995) reported a case of body rocking (*jactatio corporis nocturna*) that was successfully treated with hypnosis. At presentation the patient was a 26-year-old female with a history of rocking beginning as an infant. When she awoke during the night she would rock herself back to sleep. By late adolescence she thought the rocking had disappeared. When she married at age 24 her husband complained that her rocking kept him from falling asleep and would awaken him on occasion during the night. This increased when she breast-fed their first child. She rocked on returning to bed, resulting in her husband sleeping in a separate room. Hypnosis was induced utilizing "coin fixation." (Patients are asked to fix their eyes on a coin held between the thumb and first finger. They are instructed that after a while their fingers will become tired of holding the coin and it will slip to the floor. When it falls it is a signal to let the eyes close by themselves. There are variations of this, including placing a coin in the patient's palm with suggestions that the hand will slowly turn. There comes a moment at which the coin falls. Patients have been told that when they hear the clink of the coin striking the floor their eyes will close and they will become deeply relaxed.) Suggested imagery was of watching a television set on which the program was of her sleeping beside her husband and not rocking at any time throughout the night. She was to perform self-hypnosis prior to going to bed and at least once a day. When she returned in two weeks she reported that she was able to advance her imagery to seeing herself in bed next to her husband without having the image of a television set. Her body rocking had almost disappeared and she started sleeping in bed with her husband again without awakening him. A phone call follow-up seven months after the initiation of therapy revealed the rocking had remained in remission except for two occurrences.

Hoogduin and Hagenaars (1999) reported on a case of body rocking (*jactatio corporis nocturna*) and restless-legs symptoms whose symptoms were almost completely resolved utilizing self-monitoring, hypnosis, and self-control procedures. Their patient was a 42-year-old female with a history of rolling from one shoulder to the other dating to childhood. She reported that there had never been a night since childhood that she had not suffered from these movements. She had calcifications of both shoulders and on one occasion had dislocated her shoulder. She also experienced an irritating, tickling feeling in her legs causing her to contract her leg muscles. She had taken Tegretol and Dormicum in the past with a decrease in the rolling movement but with no change in leg movements. In the first treatment session hypnosis was performed with visualization of a place that meant relaxation to her. The aim was to obtain a state of deep relaxation which could be used later as a stimulus response intervention when she felt the sensation to start rolling. The session was recorded on an audio cassette and she was asked to practice it three times a day at home. At the next session it was found that some of the suggestions on the tape met with resistance.

New suggestions were made and self-control measures were introduced. The maximum time for her to roll was fixed at 15 minutes and her partner was recruited to assist with this. She was able to achieve a relaxed state and her symptoms improved. She also had episodes of rolling when she was awake and was asked to clasp her hands together and relax them whenever she felt the need to roll. She also had feelings of agitation and was asked to record them. When the feeling arose she was to recall the part of the hypnosis induction that relaxed her the most. She found that this technique caused her to immediately feel relaxed. The number and duration of her symptoms improved, including the leg movement. When the symptoms occurred, she was able to control them. The authors concluded that it was possible that the active factor in her treatment was the reduction of tension. They also brought up an important point which the patient mentioned as far as success of hypnotic intervention in general: she had commented that the researchers' relaxed approach to her problem and the interest they expressed was helpful.

As the above reports indicate, hypnosis can be a very effective tool for improving or resolving a variety of sleep disorders. It should be utilized along with other techniques within the therapist's field of expertise. When properly used, hypnosis is self-empowering, safe, and effective.

References

Alves, R., F. Aloe, S. Tavares, S. Vidrio, L. Yanez, R. Aquilar-Roblero, L. Rosenthal, L. Villabos, F. Fernandez-Cancino, R. Drucker-Colin, and V. Chagoya DeSanchez. 1999. "Sexual Behavior in Sleep, Sleepwalking and Possible REM Sleep Behavior Disorder: A Case Report." *Sleep Research Online: SRO* 2.3: 71–72.

American Academy of Sleep Medicine. 2005. *ICSD-2 International Classification of Sleep Disorders: Diagnostic and Coding Manual,* 2nd ed. Westchester, Il: American Academy of Sleep Medicine.

American Academy of Sleep Medicine. 2014. *ICSD-3 International Classification of Sleep Disorders: Diagnostic and Coding Manual,* 3rd ed. Westchester, Il: American Academy of Sleep Medicine.

American Psychiatric Association. 2000. *Diagnosis and Statistical Manual of Mental Disorders,* 4th ed. Washington, DC: American Psychiatric Association.

American Psychiatric Association. 2013. *Diagnosis and Statistical Manual of Mental Disorders,* 5th ed. Washington, DC: American Psychiatric Association.

Anbar, Ran D. and Molly P. Slothower. 2006. "Hypnosis for Treatment of Insomnia in School-Age Children: A Retrospective Chart Review." *BMC Pediatrics* 6: 23 (August 16).

Anderson, J. A. D., E. R. Dalton, and M. A. Basker. 1979. "Insomnia and Hypnotherapy." *Journal of the Royal Society of Medicine* 72 (October): 734–739.

Appel, Philip R. 1999. "A Hypnotically Mediated Guided Imagery Intervention for Intrusive Imagery: Creating Ground for Figure." *American Journal of Clinical Hypnosis* 41 (4): 327–335.

Bannerjee, Sanjay, Anita Srivastav, and Bhupendra M. Palan. 1993. "Hypnosis and Self-Hypnosis in the Management of Nocturnal Enuresis: A Comparative Study with Imipramine Therapy." *American Journal of Clinical Hypnosis* 36 (2): 113–118.

Bauer, Keith E. and Thomas R. McCanne. 1980. "An Hypnotic Technique for Treating Insomnia." *The International Journal of Clinical and Experimental Hypnosis* XXVIII (1): 1–5.

Becker, Philip M. 1993. "Chronic Insomnia: Outcome of Hypnotherapeutic Intervention in Six Cases." *American Journal of Clinical Hypnosis* 36 (2): 98–105.

Blanco, M. S. and A. Garay. 1995. "REM Sleep Without Muscle Atonia (RSWMA): Its Association with Other Sleep Disorders." *Sleep Research* 24: 197.

Bokey, K. 1993. "Conversion Disorder Revisited: Severe Parasomnia Discovered." *Australia and New Zealand Journal of Psychiatry* 27: 694–698.

Bonakis, A., R. S. Howard, I. O. Ebrahim, S. Merritt, and A. Williams. 2009. "REM Sleep Behavior and its Associations with Young Patients." *Sleep Medicine* 10 (6): 641–645.

Cicolin, A., A. Tribolo, A. Giordano, E. Chiarot, A. Terreni, C. Bucca, and R. Mutani. 2011. "Sexual Behaviors During Sleep Associated with Polysomnographically Confirmed Parasomnia Overlap Disorder." *Sleep Medicine* 12 (5): 523–528.

Clarke, J. H., and P. J. Reynolds. 1991. "Suggestive Hypnotherapy for Nocturnal Bruxism: A Pilot Study." *American Journal of Clinical Hypnosis* 33 (4): 248–253.

Cochrane, Gordon. 1989. "The Use of Indirect Hypnotic Suggestions for Insomnia Arising from Generalized Anxiety: A Care Report." *Americal Journal of Clinical Hypnosis* 31 (3): 199–203.

Collison, David R. 1970. "Hypnotherapy in the Management of Nocturnal Enuresis." *Medical Journal of Australia* 1 (2): 52–54.

DeLord, Vincent, Sonia Khirani, Adriana Ramirez, Erick Louis Joseph, Clotilde Gambier, Maryse Belson, Francis Gajan, and Brigitte Fauroux. 2013. "Medical Hypnosis as a Tool to Acclimatize Children to Noninvasive Positive Pressure Ventilation. A Pilot Study." *Chest* 144 (1): 87–91.

Dillahunt, D. G. 1971. *A Handbook of Therapeutic Suggestions*. Bloomingdale, Il: American Society of Clinical Hypnosis-Education and Research Foundation.

Dowd, E. Thomas. 2013. "Nocturnal Bruxism and Hypnotherapy: A Case Study." *International Journal of Clinical and Experimental Hypnosis* 61 (2): 205–218.

Dumitrascu, O., C. H. Schenck, G. Applebee, and H. Attarian. 2013. "Parasomnia Overlap Disorder: A Distinct Pathophysiologic Entity or a Variant of Rapid Eye Movement in Sleep Behavior Disorder: A Case Series." *Sleep Medicine* 14 (11): 1417–1420.

Edwards, S. D. and H. I. J. van der Spuy. 1985. "Hypnotherapy as a Treatment Enuresis." *Journal of Child Psychology and Psychiatry* 26 (1): 161–170.

Gutnik, Bruce D. and William H. Reid. 1982. "Adult Somnambulism: Two Treatment Approaches." *Nebraska Medical Journal* November: 309–312.

Hauri, Peter J., Michael H. Silber, and Bradley F. Boeve. 2007. "The Treatment of Parasomnias with Hypnosis: A 5-year Follow-Up Study." *Journal of Clinical Sleep Medicine* 3 (4): 369–373.

Hoogduin, Kees and Muriel Hagenaars. 1999. "Treatment of a Woman with Jactatio Corporis Nocturna." *Hypnos* XXVI (4): 203–208.

Hoogduin, Kees and Muriel Hagenaars. 2000. "Hypnosis in Sleep Terror Disorder." *Hypnos* XXVII (4): 180–190.

Hurwitz, Thomas D., Mark W. Mahowald, Carlos H. Schenck, Janet L. Schluter, and Scott R. Bundlie. 1991. "A Retrospective Outcome Study and Review of Hypnosis as Treatment of Adults with Sleepwalking and Sleep Terror." *Journal of Nervous and Mental Disease* 179 (4): 228–233.

Khirani, Sonia, Natacha Kadlub, Vincent DeLord, Arnaud Picard, and Brigitte Fauroux. 2013. "Nocturnal Mouthpiece Ventilation and Medical Hypnosis to Treat Severe Obstructive Sleep Apnea in a Child with Cherubism." *Pediatric Pulmonology* 48: 927–929.

Koe, G. Gerald. 1989. "Hypnotic Treatment of Sleep Terror Disorder: A Case Report." *American Journal of Clinical Hypnosis* 32 (1): 36–40.

Kohen, Daniel P., Mark W. Mahowald, and Gerald M. Rosen. 1992. "Sleep-Terror Disorder in Children: The Role of Self-Hypnosis in Management." *American Journal of Clinical Hypnosis* 34 (4): 233–243.

Kohler, W. C., P. J. Kurz, and E. A. Kohler. 2014. "A Case of Successful Use of Hypnosis in the Treatment of Parasomnia Overlap Disorder." *Behavioral Sleep Medicine* 13 (5): 349–358.

Kramer, Richard I. 1989. "The Treatment of Childhood Night Terrors Through the Use of Hypnosis – A Case Study. A Brief Communication. *The International Journal of Clinical and Experimental Hypnosis* XXXVII (1): 983–984.

Kushida, C. A., A. A. Clerk, C. M. Kirsch, J. R. Hotson, and C. Guilleminault. 1995. "Prolonged Confusion with Nocturnal Wandering Arising from NREM and REM Sleep: A Case Report." *Sleep* 18: 757–764.

Limousin, N., C. Dehais, O. Gout, F. Heran, D. Oudietto, and I. Arnulf. 2009. "A Brainstem Inflammatory Lesion Causing REM Sleep Behavior Disorder and Sleepwalking (Parasomnia Overlap Disorder)." *Sleep Medicine* 10 (9): 1059–1062.

Linden, Julie H., Anuj Bhardwaj, and Ran D. Anbar. 2006. "Hypnotically Enhanced Dreaming to Achieve Symptom Reduction: A Case Study of 11 Children and Adolescents." *American Journal of Clinical Hypnosis* 48 (4): 279–289.

Lynn, Steven Jay, Anne Malakataris, Liam Condon, Reed Maxwell, and Colleen Cleere. 2012. "Post-Traumatic Stress Disorder: Cognitive Hypnotherapy, Mindfulness, and Acceptance-Based Treatment Approaches." *American Journal of Clinical Hypnosis* 54: 311–330.

Nardi, Thomas J. 1981. "Treating Sleep Paralysis with Hypnosis." *The International Journal of Clinical and Experimental Hypnosis* XXIX (4): 356–365.

Olness, Karen. 1975. "The Use of Self-Hypnosis in the Treatment of Childhood Nocturnal Enuresis." *Clinical Pediatrics* 14 (3): 273–279.

Ortega, Deems F. 1984. "Hypnosis in the Treatment of Hypnopompic Hallucinations: A Case Report." *American Journal of Clinical Hypnosis* October: 111–113.

Reid, William H. 1975. "Treatment of Somnambulism in Military Trainees." *American Journal of Psychotherapy* 29 (1): 101–106.

Reid, William H., Iqbal Ahmed, and Charles A. Levie. 1981. "Treatment of Sleepwalking: A Controlled Study." *American Journal of Psychotherapy* XXXV (1): 27–37.

Rosenberg, Carl. 1995. "Elimination of a Rhythmic Movement Disorder with Hypnosis – A Case Report." *Sleep* 18 (7): 608–609.

Schenck, C. H. and M. Howell. 2013. "Spectrum of Rapid Eye Movement Sleep Disorder (Overlap Between Rapid Eye Movement Sleep Behavior Disorder and Other Parasomnia)." *Sleep and Biological Rhythms* 11 (l): 27–34.

Schenck, C. H., J. L. Boyd, and M. W. Mahowald. 1997. "A Parasomnia Overlap Disorder Involving Sleepwalking, Sleep Terrors, and REM Sleep Behavior Disorder in 33 Polysomnographically Confirmed Cases." *Sleep* 20: 972–981.

Somer, Eli. 1991. "Hypnotherapy in the Treatment of the Chronic Nocturnal Use of a Dental Splint Prescribed for Bruxism." *International Journal of Clinical and Experimental Hypnosis* XXXIX (3): 145–154.

Stanton, Harry E. 1989. "Hypnotic Relaxation and the Reduction of Sleep Onset Insomnia." *International Journal of Psychosomatics* 36 (1–4): 64–68.

Watkins, John G. 1987. *Hypnotherapeutic Techniques. The Practice of Clinical Hypnosis*, Vol. 1. New York: Irvington.

World Health Organization. 1979. *International Classification of Diseases*, 9th ed. Geneva: World Health Organization.

World Health Organization. 2015. *International Classification of Diseases*, 10th ed. Geneva: World Health Organization.

8 Case Studies from Dr. Kohler's Practice

Hypnosis is not a stand-alone process but is utilized along with other treatment modalities to improve the patient's health. The use of hypnosis should only be considered after a thorough medical evaluation is first conducted and if its use is felt appropriate in conjunction with other therapies. Hypnosis, like other forms of therapy, does not work for everyone. However, when utilized in the proper circumstances it can be a very effective tool for improving sleep problems. One of the positive features of hypnosis is that it is self-empowering and has no significant side-effects. The following cases demonstrate some possible hypnotherapeutic approaches, selected from the many others which might also be employed. One of the authors' hopes with this book and summary of successful personal experiences is that it will encourage others to continue the effort to find better and more effective ways to utilize hypnotherapy in treating sleep disorders.

These cases – and this book in general – are meant to stimulate interest and to motivate an even greater acceleration of the use in medicine of hypnosis and hypnotic techniques. We hope these examples will help make this valuable tool even more widely used.

Case One: A.J., 54-year-old female with a history of snoring

Medical History

At the time of her initial evaluation, A.J. was a 54-year-old female with a long history of snoring. She was referred by her primary care physician for evaluation of sleepwalking dating back only one to two months. Approximately once a week her family would find her out of her bedroom. At times she attempted to leave the house. She also tried to make coffee in the blender, although there was no definite nocturnal eating.

There was a history of occasional gastroesophageal reflux disease, sleep talking, and bruxism. There was no history of nightmares, night terrors, nocturnal enuresis, or dream enactment. Excessive daytime somnolence was present. She scored an 11 on the Epworth Sleepiness

Scale (EES). (ESS scores of 10 or more are considered indicative of significant daytime somnolence.)

She slept upright in a chair or in the corner of the couch secondary to chronic brachial plexus pain from an injury suffered five years previously. Typically she went to bed around midnight and took 1–1½ hours to fall asleep. Once asleep, she would awaken three to four times, finally getting up at 5 a.m. She rarely took a nap during the day.

Her medical history was significant for multiple retinal surgeries secondary to spontaneous retinal tears. Her medications consisted of Inderal, Neurontin, OxyContin, oxycodone, and Flexeril. She smoked 1½–2 packs of cigarettes per day. She drank two to three cups of coffee daily along with a soda, but rarely used alcohol. Her handwriting had deteriorated. She denied depression. There was no family history of sleep disorder. The patient was a nurse and had been married to her second husband for ten years.

On physical examination she was overweight with a mildly flat affect. Neck circumference was 14 inches. Posterior pharyngeal narrowing was present with tongue base enlargement, and enlargement of the uvula was present. She had a Mallampati score of II.[1]

Diagnosis

Her history and physical examination were consistent with obstructive sleep apnea with the possibility of central apnea associated with pain medication. There was evidence of insufficient sleep with sleep initiation and sleep maintenance insomnia along with sleepwalking.

A split-night polysomnogram revealed an respiratory disturbance index (RDI) of 4.3. There were 19 central apneas and two obstructive hypopneas. She had no rapid eye movement (REM) sleep. Low oxygen saturation was 81%. She was started on supplemental oxygen during the study to keep her oxygen level above 90%. She was subsequently placed on 2 L/min of oxygen at home after overnight oximetry performed at home confirmed hypoxemia.[2]

Treatment

During a follow-up visit five months later she reported that she was pleased with her overall progress. She was sleeping better and was more alert during the day. However, she continued to have episodes of sleepwalking. When she returned three weeks later for training in self-hypnosis, she reported that she had had three episodes of sleepwalking in the interim, each of which occurred between 2 and 3 a.m. During the last episode, three days previously, she tore up a paperback book. A hypnosis session was held with the patient's feet on a stool, with visual imagery induction and the post-hypnotic suggestion, "whenever your feet touch the floor you will be immediately awake." A similar repeat session was held, at which time an audio tape was made so she could practice several times per day. She returned in a week and reported no episodes of sleepwalking.

Two months later she returned to the clinic and reported that she had started sleepwalking approximately once a week. She had been taking dishes out of cupboards and putting dog food on plates without memory of the episodes. She had gained weight and was experiencing increased back pain. She continued on supplemental oxygen. She was advised to practice her hypnotherapy tape on a regular basis. She was subsequently lost to follow-up. A phone call interview four years later revealed the episodes were significantly reduced and were now occurring approximately once per month.

Summary

This case points out that the use of hypnosis was of benefit but not curative. Hypnosis improved the quality of A.J.'s life, had no side-effects, and was self-empowering. Confounding factors were her insomnia, which had improved, as well as the development of possible sleep apnea associated with weight gain which was never evaluated since she did not return for follow-up.

In the treatment of sleepwalking, hypnosis may improve or cure the motor activity, i.e., walking, but not affect the arousal. The patient may still get up, but then awaken and go back to sleep.

Case Two: R.J., a 29-year-old male with sleepwalking

Medical History

R.J. was a 29-year-old male referred by a professor of sleep medicine specifically to utilize hypnosis in the treatment of the patient's sleepwalking. He had a history of sleepwalking and possible dream enactment dating back to age nine. He had obstructive sleep apnea along with central sleep apnea which developed secondary to CPAP treatment. At the time of his initial evaluation he was utilizing adaptive servo ventilation (ASV), which controlled the obstructive and central apneas; however, two weeks later when he returned for a hypnosis session, he was utilizing a nocturnal oral dental device.[3] The patient had had one episode of sleepwalking during the previous two weeks.

Treatment

A hypnotherapy session was held with the patient's feet on a stool, with visual imagery induction and post-hypnotic suggestions for ego strengthening and the suggestion that whenever his feet touched the floor he would immediately be awakened. A second session was held during which an audio tape was made for him to listen to several times per day. When he returned in two weeks he had had no episodes of sleepwalking or possible dream enactment. He related that he was exploring alternative treatments for sleep apnea. He was advised to continue to practice his hypnotherapy tape and return in three months. He never returned. A phone call to the patient four years later revealed that he had had no evidence of sleepwalking and that his apnea was cured, possibly by a tonsillectomy with a maxillary and mandibular advancement procedure which was performed six months after his last visit.

Summary

The hypnosis most likely contributed to the resolution of the sleepwalking. However, obstructive sleep apnea can be a causal/aggravating factor for sleepwalking and treatment of the underlying apnea can also result in resolution of the sleepwalking, particularly in children. Surgical intervention is often performed for children with obstructive sleep apnea. When evaluating a child for sleepwalking who also has sleep apnea it may be prudent to delay hypnosis or other treatment for the sleepwalking until after such surgery is performed to see if the sleepwalking is still occurring.

This is another example where the patient was receptive to utilizing hypnosis as a technique to attempt to eliminate the sleepwalking; he was able to get into trance and the outcome was elimination of sleepwalking as a sole modality or in conjunction with successful treatment of his sleep apnea.

Case Three: D.R., a 12-3/12-year-old male with insomnia, sleepwalking, and nocturnal eating

Medical History

D.R. was a 12 3/12 year-old male at the time his pediatric neurologist referred him for evaluation of sleep initiation and sleep maintenance insomnia along with sleepwalking. He had a history of difficulty with sleep initiation insomnia and sleep maintenance insomnia dating back to approximately age three. His symptoms had worsened over the past year. Typically he took clonazepam, clonidine, and Abilify at 8.30 p.m. and went to bed an hour later. He fell asleep within half an hour. He would sleep for several hours then awaken, get something to eat, and return to sleep. He was awakened at 7.30 in the morning by his mother and was difficult to arouse. He occasionally awoke in the morning with a headache. He was particularly tired in the afternoon, but did not nap and did not fall asleep in class. He had difficulty concentrating on his homework. His school performance had markedly deteriorated.

He denied nightmares, night terrors, and restless-leg symptoms. There was a history of sleepwalking dating back to approximately age five which was now occurring almost on a nightly basis. He would frequently awaken in another room and on one occasion he tried to leave the house. He had no memory for these episodes, which usually occurred after 11 p.m. There was no evidence of enuresis or injury. Rare sleeptalking had been present.

A previous polysomnogram had revealed a sleep latency of 38 minutes. Sleep efficiency was 88.8%. Sleep architecture was abnormal with the absence of stage REM. There was no evidence of sleep-disordered breathing. The periodic limb movement index was mildly elevated, at 12.2.

In addition to the medication noted above he was taking Concerta during the day. There was a history of orbital cellulitis at age seven for which he was hospitalized. He had a history of premature ventricular contractions and had been evaluated by a cardiologist. His growth and development were normal. His physical and neurological examination were normal. He had been diagnosed with attention deficit hyperactivity disorder (ADHD) and was now in the sixth grade and had been getting As and Bs at the beginning of the year but was failing at the time of initial evaluation.

Treatment

Age-appropriate behavioral techniques to improve sleep were discussed with the patient and his mother – for example, use the bedroom only for sleep (no TV, or computer), do not nap during the day, eat a light snack rather than a large meal near bedtime, exercise at least four to five hours before bedtime. We also discussed the possibility of teaching D.R. self-hypnosis to treat the sleepwalking. He was placed on Mirapex 0.125 mg to treat the periodic limb movements which were demonstrated in the polysomnogram.

He returned a month later. Now he was going to bed between 8.30 and 9.30 p.m. and was asleep by 11 p.m. Occasionally he got up during the night secondary to sleepwalking and nocturnal eating. At times he was not aware of the nocturnal eating. He awoke at 7.30 a.m. and was feeling more rested. He was getting up on his own whereas previously his mother had had difficulty waking him. There were no restless-leg symptoms but he continued to kick out at night. The Abilify he had been taking was discontinued and was replaced with Risperdal. His school performance improved. His behavior on Monday through Thursday appeared to be good, but on Fridays he had a "letdown." The dose of Mirapex was increased to 0.25 mg. The possibility of teaching him self-hypnosis for sleepwalking and nocturnal eating was again discussed. The family wished to wait.

He returned 2½ months later. He continued to have episodes of sleepwalking twice or three times per week and on occasion had nocturnal eating which occurred either independently or associated with sleep-walking. His periodic limb movements had improved. School grades and behavior had also improved. He continued to have difficulty focusing and irritability in the late afternoon. On one occasion he ran away. Pros and cons of adjusting his therapy were reviewed. The possibility of teaching him self-hypnosis was again discussed.

Two weeks later his mother called me and related that D.R. was having behavior problems. A polysomnogram was performed to rule out a possible underlying sleep disorder. The polysomnogram revealed a sleep latency of 3.5 minutes, REM latency markedly prolonged at 418.5 minutes, and a sleep efficiency of 98%. Sleep architecture was abnormal, with a decrease in stage REM at 5.05%. The sleep disturbance index was 6.7. The RDI was normal at 0.14 secondary to one central apnea. The snore index was 0.41. Low oxygen saturation was satisfactory at 96%. He had no periodic leg movements. The findings were reviewed with the patient and his parents in detail and they were given a copy of the report and raw data. They reported that his sleepwalking had improved overall and he was having episodes of nocturnal eating of which he was aware. He was also having episodes of "behavioral meltdown," breaking windows and kicking down a door. Concerta was discontinued with significant improvement in behavior and scholastic progress.

He returned two months later with the report that sleepwalking was occurring two to three times per month with occasional eating during the episodes. He was in the seventh grade and had been undergoing educational evaluation. He was going to bed around 9.30 p.m. and would take up to an hour to fall asleep. Generally, he slept until 7.30 a.m., but at times would awaken at 4 or 5 a.m. His ferritin level was 34 ng/mL with a total iron of 41 ng/mL.[4]

He was started on supplemental iron with vitamin C to improve absorption. He continued on Mirapex. The patient and his family decided to have him learn self-hypnosis.

They scheduled an appointment four months later. In the interim, he was having episodes of sleepwalking approximately once a week, sometimes associated with sleep eating. He also had episodes of nocturnal eating while awake during the night. (Some patients are unable to get back to sleep unless they have something to eat.) School performance had improved but hyperactivity persisted. He was going to bed between 9 and 10 p.m. and at times was still awake at 11 p.m. Once asleep, he slept throughout the night and was getting up between 7.30 and 8 a.m. feeling tired. He did not nap during the day. There were no restless-leg symptoms and his nocturnal myoclonus/periodic limb movements had improved.

After discussing hypnosis with D.R., his mother, and grandmother, a hypnotic session was held with his feet on a stool. Visual imagery induction was carried out with post-hypnotic suggestions for ego strengthening, improved sleep, and awakening whenever his feet touched the floor. A second session was held during which time an audio tape was made. He was to practice the tape twice a day.

When he returned two weeks later he had had no episodes of sleepwalking. There was one episode of nocturnal eating of which he was aware starting 40 minutes after he went to bed. He was practicing his hypnotherapy tape on a regular basis. He was going to bed around 9 p.m. and taking approximately an hour to fall asleep. He slept throughout the night, getting up at 8 a.m. He continued to practice his hypnotherapy tape and returned in two months for follow-up.

Result

At follow-up there was no evidence of sleepwalking or nocturnal eating. There were no restless-leg symptoms or evidence of nocturnal myoclonus. His school performance and behavior had improved. He was going to bed around 9.30 p.m. and falling asleep within an hour. He slept throughout the night, getting up at 6 a.m. He was instructed to practice his hypnotherapy tape on a regular basis, follow behavioral techniques to improve sleep, and continue using Mirapex. He was subsequently lost to follow-up.

Summary

This case demonstrates a multiplicity of sleep problems, including sleepwalking, nocturnal eating with and without sleepwalking, sleep initiation and sleep maintenance insomnia, and periodic limb movement disorder. The patient also had ADHD and behavioral problems. It is well documented that poor-quality and/or insufficient sleep can lead to symptoms consistent with ADHD and problems with behavior. Improving the quality and quantity of sleep will ameliorate the ADHD symptoms and abnormal behavior. Hypnosis was utilized as a therapeutic tool in addition to behavioral techniques and medication to improve his various sleep problems. He demonstrated both types of nocturnal eating, the type associated with sleepwalking as well as sleep-related eating disorder, where a person has difficulty going back to sleep without eating. His insomnia improved with a combination of hypnosis, behavioral techniques, and medication.

Case Four: S.T., a 77-year-old female with sleepwalking

Medical History

S.T. was 77 at the time she was referred by her board-certified sleep specialist and pulmonologist for treatment of her sleepwalking. She had a history of nightmares and sleepwalking dating back 13 years. The episodes occurred in cycles of approximately three times per week followed by several weeks without any episodes, then another week or so, again with as many as three episodes per week. With one exception – when she tried to leave the house and found herself on the porch – her perambulations were inside. After the death of her husband three years earlier, sleepwalking continued. She thought that "scary dreams" awakened her. "That's why I get up and walk," she said during her initial evaluation, "I think someone is in the room with me." One of her adult daughters added that she "screams and hollers," presumably as a result of the dreams. There was no evidence of nocturnal eating, bruxism, or nocturnal enuresis. There were no reports of restless-leg symptoms. Typically she went to bed between 10 and 11 p.m. and got up at 7 a.m. feeling refreshed. Nevertheless, she reported that approximately an hour after getting up she would become tired again and would notice excessive daytime somnolence.

The review of systems was positive for heart rhythm dysfunction, chronic obstructive pulmonary disease, asthma, hypertension, acid reflux, glaucoma, arthritis, and thyroid cancer. She also had basal cell carcinoma of the face and a history of urinary tract infections. There was no history of anemia or diabetes mellitus. There had been no syncope or seizure-like activity and no evidence of depression.

Physical examination showed normal results for her age with the following two exceptions: she was blind in her right eye and her Mallampati score was high at IV. As mentioned previously, elevated Mallampati scores are an indication of potential obstructive sleep apnea. However, a previous polysomnogram revealed evidence of mild sleep-disordered breathing without definite apnea. The RDI was 0.7 with a low oxygen saturation of 89%. Sleep architecture was abnormal with only 2% of the night spent in stage REM. During the polysomnogram there were reported episodes of mild crying out and talking.

Treatment

A hypnotherapy session was held. The patient placed her feet on a stool. Visual imagery induction was carried out with post-hypnotic suggestions for her to become alert whenever her feet touched the floor. A second session was held during which time an audio tape was made. It was recommended that she practice the tape approximately twice per day and she was to call in two weeks for a progress report. During the telephone conversation she related that she was extremely pleased with the results. There had been no evidence of sleepwalking. Occasional nightmares were present. She was to gradually cut back on the use of the hypnosis tape from twice per day to once per day for a couple of weeks and then once every other day and then discontinue it. She was advised to restart use of the tape if needed. She was to follow up with her referring sleep specialist. During a follow-up phone call almost six years after the initial treatment with hypnosis, the patient and her adult daughter confirmed that there had been no evidence of sleepwalking since the initial treatment.

Summary

This is a case where the patient's compliance and her belief in the efficacy of hypnosis contributed to the success of the therapy. Another important factor was felt to be the support which she had from her daughter.

Case Five: A.R., a 16-9/12-year-old with parasomnia overlap disorder

Medical History

A.R. was a 16 9/12-year-old who was brought to the Sleep Center by his mother for evaluation of "sleep talking, and sleep running with screaming." He had had seven or more episodes of dream enactment in the previous nine months. His mother related that when he had the episodes he "barreled out of the room" and presented a danger to himself and to her. He dreamt a lizard was in his bed, and that someone was chasing him, so he got out of bed and ran. He dreamt that he was late for school and got out of bed to shower. He dreamt that thieves took over the school and he had to stop them; they drew a gun on him and began fighting so he ran from them. His mother tried to stop him and he began fighting with her, fell over some exercise equipment, and sustained a musculoskeletal injury. He also had episodes of sleepwalking occurring one to three hours after falling asleep where he would get out of bed, answer with bizarre speech, and return to bed without memory for the episodes. This was in contrast to the episodes in which he remembered the dreams and potentially acted them out.

He also had a history of sleeptalking approximately three nights a week which usually occurred two to three hours after going to sleep. He typically went to bed between 10 and 11 p.m. and fell asleep quickly. He slept throughout the night except for the episodes mentioned above. He would get out of bed at 6 a.m., feeling tired. He did not take a nap during the day and denied excessive daytime somnolence; he scored a 2 on the ESS. A.R. slept in a queen-sized bed in the supine position in his own room.

He denied awakening with a dry mouth. There were no restless-legs symptoms or evidence of nocturnal myoclonus. There was no history of nocturnal enuresis, gastroesophageal reflux disease, or deterioration of memory. There had been no cataplexy, sleep paralysis, or hypnagogic hallucinations. There was no history of snoring. He had a history of occasional night sweats.

The past medical history revealed no severe infections. There was a possible allergy to Ceclor which caused hives. He was taking no medication on a regular basis. He had had an adenoidectomy as well as his wisdom teeth removed. At age ten he was hit in the right frontal area with a metal bat without loss of consciousness. There was no history of nasal fracture. He denied the use of cigarettes, alcohol, or illicit drugs. He drank a minimal amount of caffeine.

The review of systems was negative for anemia, diabetes mellitus type 2, thyroid dysfunction, cardiac, pulmonary, or renal dysfunction. There had been no syncope or seizure-like activity. There was no history of hypertension. He denied depression. He scored a zero on the Beck Depression Inventory. At the time of his initial evaluation he was getting As in school.

The family history revealed that the patient's mother had insomnia. He had two half-brothers; one on the maternal side had several minor episodes of sleepwalking. The patient's paternal grandfather had a history of sleepwalking. The rest of the family history was unremarkable.

Diagnosis

Based on his history it was felt that A.R. had characteristics of REM sleep behavior disorder (RBD), with memory for his dreams and acting them out, which is a REM parasomnia. He also had evidence of sleepwalking, a non-REM parasomnia, with no memory for the episodes. This would fit into the category of parasomnia overlap disorder (POD), as discussed in Chapter 7.

A polysomnogram showed sleep latency was 25 minutes, REM latency was mildly shortened at 73.5 minutes, and sleep efficiency was 87%. Sleep architecture revealed that he spent 17.89% in delta sleep and 28.31% in stage REM. The RDI was 4.02 and the sleep disturbance index was 19.3. He had no episodes of snoring. Oxyhemoglobin saturation nadir was 91%. There were no periodic limb movements. He had notable intermittent loss of REM atonia on the electromyogram across all four REM episodes, but had no vocalization or abnormal movement. These findings along with his history provided evidence of RBD and sleepwalking, a non-REM parasomnia meeting criteria for POD.

Treatment

At the time he was seen in follow-up two weeks later there was no reported evidence of intervening dream enactment. He did have several episodes of sleepwalking occurring one to three hours after falling asleep, during which he got out of bed. His mother saw him and asked what he was doing and he answered with bizarre speech and returned to bed. There was no memory for the episodes, in contrast to episodes of dream enactment.

The results of the polysomnogram were discussed. His neurological examination and neurological history were unremarkable. Potential etiologic factors for RBD were discussed. It was recommended that magnetic resonance imaging (MRI) of the brain be performed.

During the visit the patient underwent a hypnosis session with his feet on a stool. Induction was by visual imagery and post-hypnotic suggestions were made for improved sleep and awakening whenever his feet would touch the floor. An audio tape of the session was made which he was asked to practice once or twice a day.

He returned for follow-up a week later but had not been able to practice hypnotherapy since his tape had malfunctioned. He reported two episodes of dream enactment. One event occurred when he and his mother were out of town in a motel; he dreamt there was something on his pillow and he jumped out of his bed and "hopped" on to his mother's bed. On another occasion he dreamt there was something in his bed and hopped out of bed. There was no evidence of definite additional sleepwalking. Another hypnotherapy was held utilizing visual imagery induction with post-hypnotic suggestions for improved sleep, ego strengthening, and the suggestion that whenever his feet would touch the floor he would immediately awaken and go back to sleep as soon as he wanted to. The session was again carried out with the patient's feet on a stool. An audio tape was made which he was asked to practice once or twice a day.

The patient's mother was called three days later to discuss the results of the MRI, which had shown a possible old lacunar infarct in the left basal ganglia. Further evaluation by a neurologist was recommended. The mother reported that he had had one episode in which he hopped out of bed and awoke as soon as he stood up. He was utilizing his hypnotherapy tape on a regular basis.

Three months later his mother called reporting that he had made significant improvement but had recent episodes of hopping out of bed and running. It was recommended that we proceed with an additional hypnotherapy tape with additional post-hypnotic suggestions. They did not follow through with an additional session.

Two months later his mother called relating that he was to go abroad the following summer and she wanted the episodes completely controlled. Approximately once a week he was getting out of bed but did not run and would talk with no awareness of the event. Several times per week he would have episodes of sleeptalking without remembrance of them. He was placed on a trial of clonazepam 0.5 mg at bedtime.

Five weeks later his mother called relating that he had been practicing his hypnotherapy tape and using 0.5 mg clonazepam at bedtime. Rare episodes were reported. On one occasion he got out of bed and stood by the bedside but did not walk. On another occasion he urinated on the wall without having memory for the episode. His clonazepam was increased to 0.75 mg.

Eleven months later he returned to the Sleep Center. There had been no episodes of sleepwalking or dream enactment over the past semester while at college. He typically was going to bed between 12.30 and 1 a.m. and falling asleep relatively quickly. He was getting up at 10 a.m. feeling refreshed. His clonazepam had been increased to 1 mg at bedtime and was continued.

The next contact was 20 months later. He had been having episodes approximately once per month where he would get out of bed and awaken as soon as his feet touched the floor. Sleeptalking had been present. There was no evidence of dream enactment. He had discontinued clonazepam because of excessive daytime somnolence. He was going to bed around 10.30 p.m. Over the past six months he had developed increasing sleep initiation insomnia, taking several hours to fall asleep, and had started taking zolpidem 5 mg at bedtime. He was getting up at 8 a.m. feeling relatively refreshed. A hypnotherapy session was held with his feet on a stool with visual imagery induction and post-hypnotic suggestions for improved sleep, ego strengthening, and a reminder that whenever his feet touched the floor he would immediately awaken. Behavioral techniques for improved sleep were discussed. He was to continue zolpidem 5 mg at bedtime as needed.

Five months later he returned to the Sleep Center. Approximately twice a month he would dream that there was something in his bed that caused him to get out of bed. However, as soon as his feet touched the floor he would be immediately awake and then would go back to sleep. He continued to experience sleep initiation and maintenance insomnia. Zolpidem 5 mg was beneficial to some degree. Behavioral techniques for improved sleep were again reviewed. He was placed on zolpidem ER 12.5 mg at bedtime.

A phone conference was held 23 months later. Episodes were occurring every four to six weeks where he would get out of bed, but would awaken as soon as his feet touched the floor. He was subsequently lost to follow-up.

Summary

This is a rare case of POD. Hypnosis was effective for the dream enactment, RBD as well as for the sleepwalking, the non-REM parasomnia. Hypnosis inhibited the motor activity but not the arousals. Clonazepam appeared to be beneficial for a period of time but had the side-effect of drowsiness and was discontinued. The zolpidem helped with his insomnia in conjunction with behavioral therapy and hypnosis. It should be noted that zolpidem has a history of causing sleepwalking in some patients.

Hypnosis was not a stand-alone therapy but was used in conjunction with other regimens.

In summary, there are a number of important lessons we can derive from the preceding cases. Hypnosis is a valuable, effective technique that can improve certain sleep disorders. It is safe, self-empowering, and relatively inexpensive. In order for hypnosis to be effective, the patient needs to believe in its potential benefit and practice the technique.

Hypnosis is not a stand-alone therapy. Similar to other therapeutic interventions, hypnosis is not effective for everyone and should be utilized in conjunction with other forms of therapy.

Hypnosis has a unique role in treating sleep disorders. The above cases would not have been effectively treated without its use.

Notes

1 A neck circumference of 15 inches or more in females or 17 inches or more in males is considered to be correlated with increased incidence of obstructive sleep apnea. Mallampati scores range from I to IV; the higher the score, the higher degree of posterior pharyngeal narrowing.
2 RDIs of 5 or more are by definition sleep apnea. An apnea is cessation of airflow for 10 seconds or more whereas a hypopnea is a decrease in airflow of 10 seconds or more followed by a lowering of oxygen or an arousal. Obstructive apnea occurs when the throat narrows and blocks the airflow. With a central apnea the signals to breathe are not generated by the brain. Potential medical complications of sleep apnea include hypertension, stroke, heart attack dementia, elevated cholesterol, elevated blood sugar, and depression. Treatment modalities include continuous positive airway pressure (CPAP), uvulopalatopharyngoplasty surgery, or a mandibular advancement device. A split-night polysomnogram is an initial baseline study performed for several hours followed by a CPAP titration if indicated by the severity of the apnea. Hypoxemia means abnormally low oxygen.
3 ASV is a type of positive airway pressure therapy that has been found to be particularly effective for central apneas. The oral dental device anchors on the upper teeth and pulls the lower jaw forward, opening the airway. Tolerance to positive airway pressure therapy varies, with reports of 20–30% of patients unable to tolerate it.
4 Ferritin is the iron-binding protein and levels below 50 have been associated with restless leg symptoms and periodic limb movement disorder.

Reference

Lynn, Steven Jan and Judith W. Rhue. 1991. *Theories of Hypnosis. Current Models and Perspectives.* New York: Guilford Press.

9 The (Very) Exciting Future

Speaking before sleep specialists from around the United States, Dr. Kohler began his presentation of August, 2014, in St. Petersburg, Florida, by exhorting them to benefit from the many advantages of using hypnosis. He encouraged them to embrace the use of hypnotic techniques and, by using them in the treatment of a great variety of sleep disorders, to join the renaissance of a field that is now increasingly recognized around the world for its solid scientific foundation.

At the time Current Concepts in Sleep 2014 was the most recent in the series of annual conferences focused on sleep medicine sponsored by a consortium of sleep centers in the Tampa Bay area that had been held every year for more than a decade. "I have a great passion for the use of hypnosis in sleep medicine," Dr. Kohler told his large audience, "and I hope I can transfer that passion to *y'all*!"

He continued by underlining the great need to have more professionals who are properly trained in this important field and who are able to use hypnosis in sleep medicine, to help meet the current increasing and unmet need. "It's a very valuable tool and, unfortunately, it's well underutilized," Dr. Kohler noted. "We need practitioners" competent in the use of this technique to help resolve many sleep problems in a manner that is more effective, safer and more cost-effective than what is commonly used today.

Dr. Kohler also addressed some of the unfounded fears and concerns that many in the general public have. "Unfortunately, hypnosis has gotten a bad rap over the years because of the various hypnotists on the stage," he said. "But it is a very valuable tool and, unlike the conception that you are under the control of the hypnotist, you are not."

He emphasized that, while undergoing hypnosis, "you are free to think, to act on your own." And added that the hypnotherapist "does not control you," although the process alters the patient's attention. In summary: "Hypnosis is altered awareness, it's focused attention, there is dissociation, suggestibility, and there is altered neuro-physiology."

Currently a significant limitation to the use of hypnosis in sleep medicine is the lack of awareness of the potential utility of this valuable technique and the lack of sleep specialists trained in hypnosis. Training can be obtained by physicians and other clinicians while continuing their current practice by attending various seminars and courses given by the American Society of Clinical Hypnosis, the Society for Clinical and Experimental Hypnosis, and the Milton H. Erickson Foundation (listed in the Resources section, Appendix D).

As the unfounded historic stigma attached to hypnosis in medicine is pushed back and as more people see it as a scientifically based therapy – that there is a measurably distinct state known as hypnosis – a greater acceptance and use of hypnotic techniques has been taking place. The authors foresee a valuable and exciting future role in this field for all practitioners. In Chapter 1 the authors have stated that hypnosis can be a non-invasive, important way in which certain sleep disorders can be treated effectively and with fewer side-effects than with other alternatives. However, to be safe and for its effective use, it is essential that the following two conditions be met: first, medical hypnosis should only be used by a fully and properly trained professional; and, second, that trained individual should only use hypnotic techniques within the person's own scope of practice. A sleep physician trained in hypnosis should not utilize the technique for, let's say, a dermatological or psychological problem unless that person also had the appropriate training in those areas or the assistance of a person properly trained in them. Even after having used hypnosis in his clinical practice for more than two decades, Dr. Kohler always limited himself to the use of hypnotic techniques to sleep medicine and to the other two medical specialties in which he was board-certified.

From the beginning one of the goals of this book has been to familiarize the sleep community with the safe and effective nature and the many benefits of using hypnosis in the treatment of sleep problems. Likewise and equally importantly, it is hoped that hypnotherapists would see the value of hypnosis in treating sleep problems and increase their knowledge of and familiarity with the many and enormously varied issues in this field that could significantly benefit from their skills.

The authors have reviewed the many reasons for the current change in perception and, as a result, are quite optimistic. What are the reasons for this optimism, for this expectation of an exciting future in sleep medicine and of a more widespread use of medical hypnosis? In summary, it is the belief that the rapid and major advances in four related fields have created an unstoppable momentum and a synergy that can only lead to even more exceptional discoveries and results. For the reasons mentioned earlier, each of these related fields is now benefitting from simultaneous discoveries and insights. This is seen most clearly in the phenomenal progress already reached in our understanding of the brain. Among the best and clearest summaries are recent works by Michio Kaku, Ph.D., a professor of theoretical physics at the City College and City University of New York, and Ray Kurzweil, Ph.D., a leading inventor, thinker, and futurist, currently Director of Engineering at Google focused on machine learning and language processing.[1]

Similar – parallel and concomitant – advances have been reached in our understanding of sleep. Dr. Hobson's major insights and detailed, yet clear, explanations related to the new sciences of sleep and dreaming seem to indicate that a better understanding of the nature and purpose of these strands is well within reach. And, as we have seen through previous chapters, hypnosis is recognized as a valid, scientifically based medical tool.

These are not the only reasons for the authors' optimism. The exciting future they see is built on three additional developments which will, in their opinion, lead to a continuation of this forward movement of discoveries and insights at an increasingly rapid pace, on a global scale.

First, as mentioned before, the development of new tools and techniques, especially in medicine. We know that the introduction of magnetic resonance imaging (MRI) machines and advanced brain scans beginning in the mid-1900s and the first decade of this century has transformed neuroscience. According to Dr. Kaku, "we have learned more about the brain in the last fifteen years than in all prior human history," and "physicists have played a pivotal role in this endeavor, providing a flood of new tools with acronyms like MRI, EEG, PET, CAT, TCM, TES, and DBS that have dramatically changed the study of the brain" (Kaku 2014, 5). Yet, much more is expected to come in the next few years. In *The Future of the Mind* Dr. Kaku describes the arrival of technologies previously considered impossible, such as videotaping our dreams, communicating telepathically, recording memories, and performing telekinesis. He then adds his predictions of what might be possible "from a physicist's perspective" in a very near future – for instance, the ability to upload our brains to a computer, neuron for neuron, or to control computers and robots with our minds. When these are superimposed on Dr. Kurzweil's predictions for computers and artificial intelligence (by 2019, a $1,000 PC will have the computing power of the human brain; by 2029, a $1,000 PC will be a thousand times more powerful than the human brain; and by 2055, $1,000 of computing power will equal the processing power of all the humans on the planet) (Kaku 2014, 271), we can begin to visualize the nature and potential impact these new techniques and tools will have on future research.

Another example directly related to sleep research is Dr. Kaku's description of how the "spectacular" success of "the first generation of brain scans" very soon will be eclipsed by what's forecast for the future. In contrast with the "thirty or so regions of the brain [that] were known with any certainty" before, "now the MRI machine alone can identify two to three hundred regions of the brain, opening up entirely new frontiers for brain science" (Kaku 2014, 31). He adds that fundamental improvements are also foreseen in the spatial and temporal resolutions of MRI machines. "The holy grail of this approach would be to create an MRI-like machine that could identify individual neurons and their connections," he adds, concluding that "no matter how spectacular the successes of the past fifteen years, then, they were just a taste of the future" (Kaku 2014, 32). Creating portable MRI devices either the size of cell phones or actually embedded in the intelligent devices can only add to their usefulness.

Second, the authors see a parallel momentum in the growth and availability of opportunities for learning and training offered to an increasingly greater number of interested students and practitioners in the health field, and specifically, in sleep medicine and hypnosis. Along these lines what is new and revolutionary in hypnosis, for instance, is that the current, more scientific, physiological basis – the ability to document this different state – is expected to lead to its acceptance by a greater number of interested practitioners, who will become more and more eager to undergo the training which is essential to its successful use.

And third, this momentum is not isolated or confined only to a few academic or research centers. It is global and interactive, fomented through modern channels of communication – formal and informal – through exchange programs and through international gatherings of unprecedented number, variety, and format.

In the field of sleep, for instance, this is evident as we look at the international source of sleep studies, at the level of global acceptance and use of sleep medicine, and at the diversity of participants in sleep seminars and conventions. The authors believe that we are only at the beginning, simply the initial stage, of greater international awareness, acceptance and use. Much is being done already beyond Europe and North America, with sleep research thriving, for instance, in Brazil and South Korea. Sergio Tufik, Ph.D., and his group have a very active research and clinical program at Universidade Federal de São Paulo and also through the Centro de Estudos do Sono (Instituto do Sono) led by Dr. Tufik, also in São Paulo. With the expanding interest we witness around the world and the modern communication and training tools available, the study of sleep will grow exponentially. The global nature of sleep research and the treatment of sleep disorders have been dramatically demonstrated during the past six World Congresses on Sleep Medicine held every two years since 2005 (Berlin, Bangkok, São Paulo, Québec, Valencia, and Seoul).

These three factors will, in the authors' opinion, have a major impact on all four areas of research mentioned at the beginning (brain, sleep, dreaming, and hypnosis). Incrementally, in only a few years, the synergy among the four will add further to the dramatic changes expected in our understanding of sleep, hypnosis, and the use of hypnotic techniques in the treatment of a broadening range of sleep disorders.

Taking a brief look at each of these component factors, it is difficult not to see the trends, the overlaps, and the consequent excitement about the future. Beginning with brain research: modern science and technology are giving us the opportunity to understand for the first time how the brain works. The new images scientists are now able to generate help us see for the first time white-matter fibers (more than 100,000 miles) and the specific pathways underlying cognitive functions. New scientific tools can document physiological changes in the brain. Individual nerve cells can be located and related to specific images seen by the eyes. Scientists are beginning to understand how information is stored (and retrieved). Full of extraordinary photographs and illustrations, a recent special issue of the *National Geographic* introduced to today's interested readers concepts perhaps unimaginable to the most sophisticated researchers a mere century ago.[2]

Eight years after the mathematician John von Neumann (1903–1957) created the architecture of our modern computer (the *von Neumann machine*), and only months before his death, he was working on a series of lectures which were posthumously published in 1958 as *The Computer and the Brain*. In a 2012 introduction to the third edition, Dr. Kurzweil called the book "the earliest serious examination of the human brain from the perspective of a mathematician and computer pioneer" (von Neumann 2012, xxiv). As early as 1957, von Neumann concluded that "the speed of neural processing is extremely slow, on the order of a hundred calculations per second, but the brain compensates for this through massive parallel processing" and that he "correctly concludes that the brain's remarkable powers come from the ten billion neurons being able to process information all at the same time" (von Neumann 2012, xxvi). In his foreword Kurzweil points out that von Neumann's estimates and forecasts are remarkable for the mid twentieth century, "given the primitive state of neuroscience at the time." Von Neumann "correctly concludes that "neurons can learn patterns from their inputs, which we now know are coded in neurotransmitter concentrations," but what only became known much more recently is that "learning also takes place through the creation and destruction of connections between neurons." He adds:

> The reality is that we remember only a very small fraction of our thoughts and experiences, and these memories are not stored as bit patterns at a low level (such as a video image), but rather as sequences of higher-level patterns. Our cortex is organized as a hierarchy of pattern recognizers.
>
> (von Neumann 2012, xxvii)

In a chapter of *How to Create a Mind* (Kurzweil 2012), titled "The Law of Accelerating Returns Applied to the Brain," Dr. Kurzweil summarizes the astonishing changes he predicts will take place in brain research during the next few years and decades. "Progress in medicine has historically been based on accidental discoveries, so progress during the earlier era was linear, not exponential," he explains. "With the gathering of the software of life – the genome – medicine and human biology have become an information technology" and this will continue its growth at an exponential progression (Kurzweil 2012, 252). "Brain scanning technologies are improving in resolution, spatial and temporal, at an exponential rate," he writes, adding that "different types of brain scanning methods being pursued range from completely noninvasive methods that can be used with humans to more invasive or destructive methods on animals" (Kurzweil 2012, 262).

Today the new research being conducted in locations such as the Allen Institute for Brain Science in Seattle and by neuroscientist and psychiatrist Karl Deisseroth and his colleagues at Stanford is also expected to shed much additional light on our understanding of the related fields of sleep, dreaming, and hypnosis. In addition to sophisticated equipment, the methods used rely on imagination and creativity. For instance, working with thin sections of mouse brain, Dr. Deisseroth "came up with a recipe to replace the light-scattering compounds in the brain with transparent molecules." A transparent brain allows its in-depth examination "while the organ is still intact." The researchers can then "douse the brain with glowing chemical labels that latch on to only certain proteins or trace a specific pathway connecting neurons in distant regions of the brain" (Zimmer 2014, 51). Dubbed CLARITY, through this process the scientists "can then wash out one set of chemicals and add another that reveals the location and structure of a different type of neuron – in effect untangling the Gordian knot of neural circuits one by one." Similar articles describing numerous similar research projects are available in *Scientific American* and, of course, in specialized professional scientific journals.

This excitement also comes from the almost immediate global reach of such research. One of many examples comes to us from the Allen Institute, where scientists are mapping human brains donated by the families of recently deceased people by "charting the activity of 20,000 protein-coding genes at 700 sites within each brain." The scientists "estimate that 84 percent of all the genes in our DNA become active somewhere in the adult brain" (Zimmer 2014, 43). All this information is posted online, making it available for researchers worldwide, for use in conjunction with their own studies or research. Evidence of important results directly related to such newly posted information usually begins to be seen very soon after postings.

Such instant access and rapid dissemination generate further excitement through the almost daily flow of news also related to the accelerated pace of research taking place. A recent and by no means unique example is the story of how the general public as well as many interested medical professionals learned about research results announced during 2013 at the University of Rochester in New York by neurosurgeon Maiken Nedergaard and her colleagues.

In "Sleep Drives Metabolite Clearance from the Adult Brain," published in *Science*,[3] lead authors Lulu Xie and Hongyi Kang describe results that appear to suggest that during sleep the brain cleans itself. According to Emily Underwood, also writing in *Science* (2013, 301), the new study provides what "Charles Czeisler, a sleep researcher at Harvard Medical School in Boston, calls the 'first direct experimental evidence at the molecular level' for what could be sleep's basic purpose: It clears the brain of toxic metabolic byproducts." The Editor's Summary in *Science* states that:

> Using state-of-the-art in vivo two-photon imaging to directly compare two arousal states in the same mouse, Xie *et al.* (p. 373; see the Perspective by Herculano-Houzel) found that metabolic waste products of neural activity were cleared out of the sleeping brain at a faster rate than during the awake state. This finding suggests a mechanistic explanation for how sleep serves a restorative function, in addition to its well-described effects on memory consolidation.
>
> (Xie et al. 2013, 373)

In an interview disseminated by the University of Rochester Dr. Nedergaard explained that the "study shows that the brain has different functional states when asleep and when awake." Dr. Nedergaard, co-director of the University's Center for Translational Neuromedicine, added that "in fact, the restorative nature of sleep appears to be the result of the active clearance of the by-products of neural activity that accumulate during wakefulness." In other words, according to the University of Rochester, "in findings that give fresh meaning to the old adage that a good night's sleep clears the mind, a new study shows that a recently discovered system that flushes waste from the brain is primarily active during sleep."

Within days, there were hundreds – possibly thousands – of reports on television, newspapers, internet blog reports, and interviews posted around the world in many languages. "Sleep 'cleans' the brain of toxins," according to the BBC. "A good night's sleep scrubs your brain clean, researchers find," announced NBC. The National Public Radio had a feature about how "Brains Sweep Themselves Clean of Toxins during Sleep." And, according to the *Washington Post*'s lead sentence, "While we are asleep, our bodies may be resting, but our brains are busy taking out the trash."[4] Why was this important? In simple language the article explained:

> "Sleep puts the brain in another state where we clean out all the byproducts of activity during the daytime," said study author and University of Rochester neurosurgeon Maiken Nedergaard. Those

byproducts include beta-amyloid protein, clumps of which form plaques found in the brains of Alzheimer's patients.

Staying up all night could prevent the brain from getting rid of these toxins as efficiently, and explain why sleep deprivation has such strong and immediate consequences. Too little sleep causes mental fog, crankiness, and increased risks of migraine and seizure. Rats deprived of all sleep die within weeks.

(Kim 2013, 373)

All this happened within a few days of the initial publication in the scientific journal. Such detailed and rapid circulation of new scientific findings has enormous implications for the advancement of the new sciences of the brain, of sleep, and, of course, hypnosis. This was also an example of the kind of sleep research that could not have been done just a few decades ago. Underwood describes how, during the preceding two years, mice were trained "to relax and fall asleep on a two-photon microscope, which can image the movement of dye through living tissue" (Underwood 2013, 301). The kind of ingenuity and creativity shown in devising and carrying out this study has been present among extraordinary scientists throughout history. However, the range of modern tools available today, added to the rapid, global exchange and dissemination of information, are two of the new and major factors that create such high expectations for the future of research in fields such as sleep and hypnosis.

Another focus which has led research in these areas towards new, unexpected directions is the study of the brain and of the sleep patterns and habits of birds, dolphins, and other animals that have not been examined before with the new techniques now available. The subsequent scientific as well as popular articles have also been synergistic and a growing field. A good example is the story of Chaser, a border collie at times called "the smartest dog in the world."[5] John Pilley, a retired psychology professor, has devoted up to five hours a day, five days a week for more than nine years to teaching words and word recognition to Chaser. As a result, according to Pilley, Chaser now has three times the vocabulary of a two-year-old toddler and correctly identifies "95 percent or more" of a thousand toys when called out by Pilley. Brian Hare, an evolutionary anthropologist at Duke University, "believes Chaser is the most important dog in the history of modern scientific research" because of his use of social inference – he is "using the same ability that kids use when they learn lots of words." And this, according to Hare, is not only important but, surprisingly, a very new finding. "There was no evidence until the last decade that dogs were capable of inferential reasoning, absolutely not," he said on the CBS *60 Minutes* documentary aired October 5, 2014. "So that's what's new, that's what's shocking, that of all the species, it's dogs that are showing a couple of abilities that are really important that allow humans to develop culture and language."

Added to this example of new research is the specific way – impossible only a few decades ago – in which such research is conducted. According to the CBS documentary, Dr. Greg Berns, a physician and neuroscientist at Emory University, "has studied the human brain for more than two decades, but three years ago questions he had about his own dog inspired him to start looking at the canine brain." He began to use functional MRI (fMRI) machines, conducting brain scans on dogs that were awake and not sedated. The resulting "slicing" enables Dr. Berns to see which parts of the brain respond to different signals. One significant finding, Dr. Berns believes, is that he now has evidence that, through their scent, dogs are able to recognize "somebody extremely important to them." When the dogs were exposed to cotton swabs with different scents, no matter what the scent was, an area right behind the nose was activated. However, when the scent was that of their owner's sweat, "another area of the brain was stimulated – the caudate nucleus, or 'reward center'." This, according to Dr. Berns, is "the same area in a human brain that activates when we listen to a favorite song or anticipate being with someone we love."

These kinds of remarkable recent findings, made possible through the use of modern tools and techniques, so far have multiplied most rapidly in the fields of brain study and of sleep. The pace of research continues to expand. Examples are The Human Brain Project being funded by the European Union and, in the United States, new federal funding has been announced recently by the Brain Research through Advancing Innovative Neurotechnolgies (BRAIN) an initiative through which various consortia have also announced their partnerships and funding plans. For instance, six projects selected at the University of California, Berkeley, focus specifically on mapping and studying the brain. They include the study of acousto-optic waveguides researching a way to channel light deeper to probe cell-to-cell signaling in the brain; the probing of cell-to-cell communication in the brain using novel nanocrystals; and the development of instrumentation and computational methods by achieving an increase in the density and electronic sophistication of recording arrays.[6]

Another example of how modern brain research can lead to unexpected results is the story of the three recipients of the 2014 Nobel Prize in Medicine. According to the Nobel Committee, in 1971 New York-born researcher John O'Keefe discovered a "positioning system" (an "inner GPS") in the brain of rats. He found that a type of nerve cell in the hippocampus was always activated when a rat was at a certain place in a room, while other nerve cells were activated when the rat was at other places. O'Keefe called them "place cells" and concluded that they formed a map of the room. But this only became truly significant decades later, in 2005, when Edvard and May-Britt Moser discovered another key component of the brain's positioning system. According to the Nobel Committee, the Norwegian husband-and-wife team "identified another type of nerve cell, which they called 'grid cells,' that generate a coordinate system and allow for precise positioning and path-finding." Working more than 30 years apart, the three recipients of the Nobel Prize "have solved a problem that has occupied philosophers and scientists for centuries – how does the brain create a map of the space surrounding us and how can we navigate our way through a complex environment?"

Foremost among the scientists who have best described the meaning and impact of such discoveries, particularly in the fields of sleep and dream research, is Harvard's Dr. Allan Hobson. In his books and scientific articles he has presented in great detail his theories and conclusions related to sleep and to what he has called this new science of brain and the new science of dreaming.

A Professor of Psychiatry, Emeritus, at Harvard Medical School, Dr. Hobson has devoted much of his life to the study of dreams based on solid neurobiological research. He has concluded that dreams are psychological phenomena resulting from specific brain activity at the cellular and molecular levels. His "brain-based approach to dreaming" is described in *The Dreaming Brain* and summarizes "the discoveries of modern sleep and dream research which have both provided the building blocks" of his integrated brain–mind theory of dreaming "and vindicated the original philosophical convictions of Ramón y Cajal and Freud" (Hobson 1988, 19). In Part IV of this work, Dr. Hobson presents his "formal analysis of dreaming inspired by the activation-synthesis hypothesis" which he has continued to develop since then, challenging Freud's theories of dream interpretation.

From Angels to Neurones: Art and the New Science of Dreaming is Dr. Hobson's collaborative work with Hellmut Wohl, an art historian whose focus includes the Renaissance and Modern periods. Their beautiful and substantive study has as its *leitmotif* their "aim of demonstrating the consilience of art and science." This they did elegantly through a historic and scientific study of the science of dreaming, illustrated with exceptionally well-chosen works of art as well as modern scientific images, such as a photomicrograph of neurones.

It is beyond the purpose of this chapter to discuss Dr. Hobson's theories in detail. His *Dreaming: An Introduction to the Science of Sleep* (2002) and *The Dream Drugstore: Chemically Altered States of Consciousness* (2001) are enjoyable, informative, and superb studies of the nature and function of dreaming, but also reflecting in detail scientific findings through which dreams can be shown to intersect and overlap with sleep and hypnosis. The central thesis of *The Dream Drugstore* is "that altered states of consciousness are the subjective concomitants of altered states of brain physiology" (Hobson 2001, 19). This work also summarizes Dr. Hobson's AIM state-space model, named after its three parameters: activation (A); input–output gating (I); and chemical modulation (or mode, M) (Hobson 2001, 45). Through several tables the reader is given a clear statement of three behavioral states in humans, the states of waking, non-rapid eye movement (NREM) sleep, and REM sleep (Hobson 2001, 52). Finally, the work also discusses the neuroimaging of hypnosis and describes a fascinating case study in which the participants were Aldous Huxley and Milton Erickson. In conclusion,

> The result of all this new work is that an objective comparative neurophysiology of altered states of consciousness is in the making. As the technology of brain imaging continues to improve and the number of studies using this exciting approach grows, it will become more and more important to characterize the conscious experience, the motivation, and the intentions of the experimental subjects.
>
> (Hobson 2001, 104)

And "now hypnosis – and related practices like relaxation and meditation – are becoming more widely accepted and lending themselves to scientific study to determine their underlying brain mechanism."

Nevertheless, there are many who go beyond Dr. Hobson's strict physiological conclusions. According to Dr. Hobson, one of the main functions of REM sleep is to "tune up" the brain for the day's work. Psychiatrist Prudence Gourguechon goes even further.[7] She writes:

> Personally, I feel so done with the idea that we have to figure out if something is psychological or physiological. If it has meaning or it is neurons firing. If the brain is tuning up to run, or processing from the day before. It doesn't have to be one or the other. It's nature AND nurture, brain AND mind, physiology AND psychology. Researchers interested in the interface between psychoanalysis and neuroscience have begun to locate, on fMRI, things like transference, empathy, affective regulation. I am excited about the possibilities that lie ahead to integrate meaning making and psychological development with new discoveries about brain function.

It is well known that Carl Gustav Jung experienced significant dreams and visions from an early age. Beginning with his university days in Basel, Jung immersed himself in the serious study of dreams, including the various phenomena that may occur during periods of hypnagogia – such as fantasies, lucid dreaming, and hallucinations. Through his writings (Jung 1989) we know that many of these dreams were self-induced and possibly the result of a concentrated technique that became known as *active imagination*. For 16 years, beginning in 1913, Jung created an encyclopedic collection and illustration of his dreams and fantasies. More than 50 exquisite colored works, painted by Jung on paper in gold and multicolored ink, were assembled in a large, red leather- bound book he called *Liber Novus,* which became known eventually as *The Red Book*. In the manuscript itself, Jung wrote in 1957:

The years, of which I have spoken to you, when I pursued the inner images, were the most important time of my life. Everything else is to be derived from this. It began at that time, and the later details hardly matter anymore. My entire life consisted in elaborating what had burst forth from the unconscious and flooded me like an enigmatic stream and threatened to break me.[8]

For several reasons this most important work was kept from the general public by Jung's family and heirs. Only in May 2000 was it released for publication through a lavish, facsimile version published in 2009. *The Red Book* – surrounded by the careful digital reproduction of many

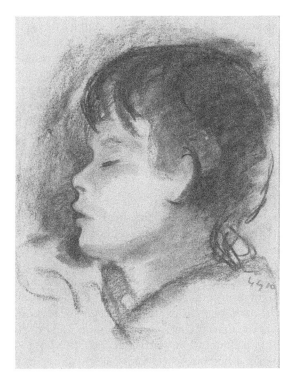

Figure 9.1 "Péter Dreaming," by János Antal Kürz. Dreams and dreaming are most often envisioned as – somehow – associated with sleep and, perhaps, with the future or with life beyond death . . . an after-life. For millennia, artists, poets and writers have attempted to portray dreams as visions and, often, as messages. Today new tools have led to new insights into the nature and purpose of dreaming. One new approach to these visions and interpretations is offered by the psychiatrist, Professor J. Allan Hobson, M.D. Among his most recent and fascinating works are *From Angels to Neurones: Art and the New Science of Dreaming* (2005) and *Psychodynamic Neurology: Dreams, Consciousness, and Virtual Reality* (2015).

of its images – was one of the two centerpieces featured at the 2013 Venice Biennale. According to Massimiliano Gioni, the exhibition's curator, "Jung sought to show 'primordial images' that are 'capable of speaking a thousand voices, the images that are capable of combining a personal destiny with a collective one'."[9] Until the last few decades sleep and dreaming could be observed, analyzed, and described. But only the images created by poets, writers, and artists could attempt to "show" – indirectly – "sleep" or "dreaming." Such mental, dream images and their representations through art and literature have been the only "documentation" available to humanity. Only now do we have the tools needed for the next, exponential leap in our understanding and in-depth scientific describing of sleep and dreaming.

Dr. Kaku illustrates the importance of modern tools in today's sleep and dream research through a series of fascinating examples from current work in several laboratories. He points out that "only in the last decade or so" have scientists been able to make significant scientific progress in their understanding of dreaming. "In fact," he notes, "scientists can now do something once considered impossible: they are able to take rough photographs and videotapes of dreams with MRI machines" and "one day, you may be able to view a video of the dream you had the previous night and gain insight into your own subconscious mind" (Kaku 2014, 171). Another astonishing new area of investigation explores the phenomenon of lucid dreaming (dreaming while you are conscious). Dr. Kaku explains it as follows:

> Brain scans of lucid dreamers show that this phenomenon is real; during REM sleep, their dorsolateral prefrontal cortex, which is usually dormant when a normal person dreams, is active, indicating that the person is partially conscious while dreaming. In fact, the more lucid the dream, the more active the dorsolateral prefrontal cortex. Since the dorsolateral prefrontal cortex represents the conscious part of the brain, the dreamer must be aware while he or she is dreaming.
>
> Dr. Hobson told me that anyone can learn to do lucid dreaming by practicing certain techniques. In particular, people who do lucid dreaming should keep a notebook of dreams. Before going to sleep, they should remind themselves that they will "wake up" in the middle of the dream and realize that they are moving in a dream world.
> (Kaku 2014, 177)

This optimism and excitement about "the possibilities that lie ahead" are equally applicable to hypnosis. As reviewed in previous chapters, the concept of what hypnosis "is" has changed from that of magic incantation to suggestion and focused attention. Current concepts now include acceptance of solid, scientific evidence of underlying changes in the brain's neural function. Theoretical differences in viewpoints continue as scientific research as well as different perspectives continue the search for an ever better understanding. In *Theories of Hypnosis: Current Models and Perspectives* the editors assembled a selection of 20 essays by leading proponents of many of these findings and overlapping theories (Lynn and Rhue 1991, 13). They called their categorical scheme "a heuristic framework for organizing theories of hypnosis," within which a broad range of hypnosis-related topics were discussed (such as hypnotic communication, the possibility that hypnotizability is plastic or modifiable, and issues related to self-deception). Overall, the contributors were asked to focus on "(1) Is hypnosis an altered state of consciousness? (2) Is hypnotic behavior involuntary? (3) How stable, trait-like, and modifiable is hypnotizability?" (Lynn and Rhue 1991, 14).

A related and very important question is: How is hypnosis and how are various theories of hypnotic behavior placed "within the larger arena of contemporary psychology" and how do they "draw on concepts from this larger domain to buttress their arguments"? (Lynn and Rhue 1991, 14). Rossi's point of view (mentioned in Chapter 4) is that there is an extensive overlap of what is today called "hypnosis" and a great number of other related, perhaps similar, approaches and theories which are today known by a different label (Rossi and Rossi 2006). Can Jung's 16-year pursuit of "the inner images" through a method he called "active imagination" be a form of autohypnosis? Is the American psychologist Mihaly Csikszentmihalyi's state of consciousness, known as *flow*, a result of focused attention or some other combination of behavior somehow, perhaps, related to hypnosis?[10]

Does American psychologist Martin E.P. Seligman's new science of Positive Pscyhology overlap with certain aspects of focused attention and autohypnosis? Dr. Seligman is professor of psychology and director of the Positive Psychology Center of the University of Pennsylvania, where he has taught for almost 50 years. Is it possible that the focus on "positive emotion" as a gateway to mental health and happiness has within it many of the elements that are also important in the use of hypnotic techniques? In one of his recent statements Dr. Seligman pointed out (in collaboration with Darwin Labarthe) that Positive Psychology has morphed into Positive Health, Positive Neuroscience, Positive Education, and the study of imagination and creativity.[11]

This evolution of our knowledge is continuing at a rapid pace. Clinical and basic research in the fields of brain function, sleep, dreaming, and hypnosis is being carried out at major academic and research centers throughout the world. The interaction of the knowledge of how the brain works, our knowledge of sleep, and our better understanding of hypnosis are developing on parallel planes that are mutually interactive and reinforcing. Today hypnosis is generally accepted as an effective tool that can be utilized by health practitioners to improve sleep and the future potential for the use of hypnosis in exploring the mind is truly exciting. Hypnosis and posthypnotic suggestions can be utilized with newer imaging techniques to explore brain mechanisms and reciprocally study the underlying tenets of hypnosis. As new techniques are developed and tested, the use of hypnosis will continue to evolve. For instance, the Rapid Reintegration Procedure developed by Edgar Barnett is such a technique, one that has been successfully utilized in delivering effective psychotherapeutic treatment for many patients. (See Barnett and Tkach 2005, for an excellent review.) Dr. Kohler believes that hypnosis may in the future provide a way to assist at least some patients with sleep apnea, eliminating their need for continuous positive airway pressure or other, more intrusive, treatment.

As summarized in Chapter 4, Dr. Bertrand Piccard's preparation for his entirely solar-powered flight around the world had already included extensive and fruitful research and experiments in sleep. On his website (www.bertrandpiccard.com) he also explained his reliance on advanced techniques of hypnosis – including autohypnosis – particularly during solar-powered flights that can only carry one pilot and consist of long flight sectors. "How can you stay alert enough to fly an airplane for five days and nights?" he asks. Dr. Piccard decided to experiment with autohypnosis. "By self-inducing a state of trance, the pilot can dissociate mind from body and so continue to concentrate on the instruments and controls even when he is resting," he explained. In Chapter 4 we mentioned that Dr. Piccard conducted a successful 72-hour simulated crossing of the Atlantic without leaving Dübendorf, Switzerland, while surrounded by medical doctors and a team of other experts, including fellow qualified practitioners of medical hypnosis who are part of his Solar Impulse project team. He observed on his website that "seeing so many doctors around Solar Im*pulse* reminded me of my first profession, although this time around I was the patient." Relying on his skills as a hypnotherapist, Dr. Piccard logged 35 rest periods of perhaps 20 minutes each during the three-day simulation.

These and other experiments were the precursors of the methodology which enabled Dr. Piccard and André Borschberg successfully to complete on July 26, 2016, the first ever circumnavigation of the Earth with a solar airplane.

Flying around the world for, at times, stretches as long as four and five consecutive days and nights, with the pilot alone at the controls while encapsulated in a 3.8 cubic meter cockpit, presented a unique human challenge. For Dr. Piccard, the use of hypnosis and hypnotic techniques provided the solution needed to cross the Atlantic Ocean and, later, the Mediterranean Sea.

We have learned from Dr. Piccard's work with hypnosis and autohypnosis that hypnotic techniques can be utilized to improve our function in a wide range of activities and situations. By allowing us to take short naps, perhaps hypnosis can provide a way to compensate for lost sleep, help with travel across time zones, or improve safety during shift work. Beyond the treatment of sleep disorders, the more such experiments are carried out, the more we will learn how hypnosis can be a tool in the study of brain function, of sleep and, in short, how it can become instrumental in improving our lives and safety. With the increased recognition of hypnosis as an effective and desirable tool for the treatment of sleep disorders its future must be considered bright.

In 2005, Arreed Barabasz wrote: "times are better now for clinicians and researchers interested in hypnosis" (Barabasz and Watkins 2005, 10). There are more courses and many ways to "specialize in this area and retain professional acceptance." He mentions that his own "appointment at Harvard Medical School and early promotion to associate professor was made possible only" because of his work in hypnosis and adds that "similar acceptance and career rewards" have come to many of his former Ph.D. students.

Dr. Barabasz discusses the need for a much greater use of medical hypnosis and notes that opportunities for training in hypnosis have increased enormously during the past decades. "At long last, hypnosis has largely overcome the prejudices in the medical profession and academia," he writes. "Hypnosis is accepted as a legitimate scientific and treatment modality" (Barabasz and Watkins 2005, 23). He cites several programs which have been in existence since the 1970s and 1980s and then mentions many of the best-known, more recent additions. For instance, there is the program at Washington State University at Pullman, where "a four-credit-hour course in clinical and experimental hypnosis has been a regular yearly part of graduate training for counseling psychologists for the past 20 years" (Barabasz and Watkins 2005, xii). Also the University of Montana at Missoula, where "a course in hypnotherapy has been a regular part of doctoral training in the APA [American Psychological Association]-accredited clinical psychology program for more than 30 years." Additional programs have been added more recently and are now available throughout the country at various levels and numerous locations, from "an increasing number of medical schools and graduate departments of psychology and counseling psychology" at the larger universities now offering training in hypnosis (Barabasz and Watkins 2005, 23). At Harvard University Medical School "hypnosis is the standard non-pharmacologic analgesia for interventional radiological procedures" (Barabasz and Watkins 2005, 23), at Stanford University Medical School "hypnosis is routinely used to prolong life and provide cancer pain relief" (Barabasz and Watkins 2005, 24), and at the University of California (Davis) Medical Center, "hypnosis is in regular use to reduce blood loss and speed healing in spinal surgery patients" (Barabasz and Watkins 2005, 24).

Medical hypnosis and the use of hypnotic techniques in medicine may now be at a stage similar to that of psychology, as was described in 2008 by Dr. Martin Seligman, in his often-cited and much-admired TED presentation titled "The New Era of Positive Psychology"[12] Apparently he was asked for a one-word summary of "the state of psychology today." He replied: "Good." Not satisfied, the interviewer requested a somewhat longer – two-word – sound bite. "The state of psychology today?" The new answer: "Not good." Well . . . "in three words?" she asked again. Professor Seligman's summary and his evaluation became "not good enough."[13]

The authors believe that the current relationship of hypnosis and sleep medicine can be seen as "good" or "not good" but more likely it's simply "not good enough." (At this time!) The increased acceptance of hypnosis by the medical profession – globally – and the cornucopia of desirable features it offers to those who use it properly promise practitioners of hypnosis and their patients a very exciting future.

Notes

1 The theoretical physicist Dr. Michio Kaku is a co-founder of String Field Theory. He is also the author of numerous books, host of science programs on radio and television, and a popular speaker. Currently he is a professor of theoretical physics at the City College and City University of New York. Additional details of his many activities can be found on his website (www.mkaku.org), which also includes details of eight books he wrote since 1994 and, in several cases, updates. Through *The Future of the Mind* (2014), Dr. Kaku conveys to his readers his views of the remarkable future in the fields of brain and dream research and addresses major issues related to the mind, consciousness, memory, and thought. Dr. Kaku's Facebook Fan Page is "an online community of over 2 million fans of *The Future of the Mind* featuring interviews," events, and presentations.

Raymond "Ray" Kurzweil, Ph.D., is an American author, computer scientist, inventor, and futurist. He is currently director of engineering at Google. After earning a B.S. in computer science and literature at the Massachusetts Institute of Technology (1970), he continued his career as an inventor, entrepreneur, and author.

From http://www.kurzweiltech.com/aboutray.html:

Kurzweil was the principal inventor of the first CCD flat-bed scanner, the first omni-font optical character recognition, the first print-to-speech reading machine for the blind, the first text-to-speech synthesizer, the first music synthesizer capable of recreating the grand piano and other orchestral instruments, and the first commercially marketed large-vocabulary speech recognition . . . . Among Kurzweil's many honors, he is the recipient of the National Medal of Technology, was inducted into the National Inventors Hall of Fame, holds twenty honorary Doctorates, and honors from three U.S. presidents.

An excellent overview of his many companies can be found on http://www.kurzeiltech.com/ktiflash.html. Also, from Kurzweil's official website (kurzweilAI.net):

Ray Kurzweil's book, *The Singularity Is Near*, was a *New York Times* bestseller, and has been the #1 book on Amazon in both science and philosophy. His latest *New York Times* bestseller is *How to Create a Mind:*

The Secret of Human Thought Revealed. His website, KurzweilAI.net, tracks daily breakthroughs in science and technology and has over three million new readers annually. In 2012, Ray Kurzweil was appointed a Director of Engineering at Google, heading up a team developing machine intelligence and natural language understanding.

2 "Secrets of the Brain" is the cover article in the February, 2014, issue of the *National Geographic* magazine (pages 21–57). It is only one among many that have been published with increasing frequency about the topics discussed in this book. The quality, clarity, and beauty of the color photographs and illustrations make this collaboration by writer Carl Zimmer and photographer Robert Clark particularly informative and enjoyable.

Not directly related to the *National Geographic* cover article, but very much to its topic, are the following additional observations by Kurzweil, especially when he describes how von Neumann perceived "the differences and similarities between the computer and the human brain."

In addition to the quotes from *The Computer and the Brain* (von Neumann 2012), the following, from Kurzweil's "Foreword to the Third Edition" (von Neumann 2012, xxv), gives us additional glimpses of John von Neumann's genius (writing before his death in 1957!): "the von Neumann machine . . . has remained the core structure of essentially every computer for the past sixty-six years, from the microcontroller in your washing machine to the largest supercomputers" (von Neumann 2012, xx).

And:

> Von Neumann starts by articulating the differences and similarities between the computer and the human brain. Given that he wrote in 1955 and 1956, the manuscript is remarkably accurate, especially in the details that are pertinent to the comparison. He notes that the output of neurons is digital: an axon either fires or it doesn't. This was far from obvious at the time, in that the output could have been an analog signal. The processing in the dendrites leading into a neuron and in the soma neuron cell body, however, are analog. He describes these calculations as a weighted sum of inputs with a threshold. This model of how neurons work led to the field of connectionism, in which systems are built based on this neuron model in both hardware and software.
>
> (von Neumann 2012, xxv)

Finally, Kurzweil predicts:

> Today the first supercomputers are being built that achieve a speed matching some of the more conservative estimates of the speed required to functionally simulate the human brain (about 10 to the 16th operations per second). I estimate that the hardware for this level of computation will cost $1,000 early in the 2020s.
>
> (von Neumann 2012, xxx)

3 *Science,* vol. 342, 18 October, 2013, includes the text of the original article by Xie et al. ("Sleep Drives Metabolite Clearance from the Adult Brain," from page 373) as well as several related essays and commentaries. In addition to the quotes included in Chapter 9, for easy reference the authors include below the abstract and the full quote from Emily Underwood ("Sleep: The Brain's Housekeeper?", page 301), describing the experiment in lay terms. Perhaps these excerpts will encourage some readers also to enjoy the original article by Xie et al.

Xie, Lulu, Hongyi Kang, Qiwu Xu, Michael J. Chen, Yonghong Liao, Meenakshisundaram Thiyagarajan, John O'Donnell, Daniel J. Christensen, Charles Nicholson, Jeffrey J. Iliff, Takahiro Takano, Rashid Deane, Maiken Nedergaard. 2013. "Sleep Drives Metabolite Clearance from the Adult Brain." *Science* 342 (6156): 373–377

Abstract

The conservation of sleep across all animal species suggests that sleep serves a vital function. We here report that sleep has a critical function in ensuring metabolic homeostasis. Using real-time assessments of tetramethylammonium diffusion and two-photon imaging in live mice, we show that natural sleep or anesthesia are associated with a 60% increase in the interstitial space, resulting in a striking increase in convective exchange of cerebrospinal fluid with interstitial fluid. In turn, convective fluxes of interstitial fluid increased the rate of β-amyloid clearance during sleep. Thus, the restorative function of sleep may be a consequence of the enhanced removal of potentially neurotoxic waste products that accumulate in the awake central nervous system.

From Emily Underwood's "Sleep: The Brain's Housekeeper?":

Once Xie was sure the mice were asleep, based on their EEG [electro-encephalogram] brain activity, she injected a green dye into their CSF [cerebrospinal fluid] through a catheterlike device in their necks. After half an hour, she awakened them by touching their tails and injected a red dye that the two-photon micsroscope could easily distinguish from the green. By tracking the movements of red and green dye throughout the brain, the team found that large amounts of CSF flowed into the brain during sleep, but not during the awake state, Nedergaard says.

A comparison of the volume of space between nerve cells while the mice were awake and asleep revealed that the glial channels carrying CSF expanded by 60% when the mice were asleep. The team also injected labeled B amyloid proteins into the brains of sleeping mice and awake mice and found that during sleep, CSF cleared away this "dirt" outside of the cells twice as quickly – "like a dishwasher," Nedergaard says. Such proteins can aggregate as pathogenic plaques inside cells and are associated with Alzheimer's disease, she says.

On pages 316–317 of the same issue of *Science* is also a Perspective/ Neuroscience essay by Suzana Herculano-Houzel ("Sleep It Out,") related to Xie et al.

The quotes in the text were downloaded from www.sciencemag.org on November 6, 2013. The quotes in Note 2 were accessed through the same link on October 10, 2014.

4 The *Washington Post*, "Brains Flush Toxic Waste in Sleep, Including Alzheimer's-Linked Protein, Study of Mice Finds," by Meeri Kim, October 19, 2013.
5 "The Smartest Dog in the World" aired on CBS *60 Minutes* on October 5, 2014. Anderson Cooper is the correspondent. Denise Schrier Cetta, producer.
    A video link can be accessed through: http://www.cbsnews.com/news/ how-smart-is-your-dog-60-minutes/. A full, illustrated transcript is available through: http://www.cbsnews.com/news/the-smartest-dog-in-the-world/.

"Inside Animal Minds" covers a wider range of reports about research on animal brains through three segments: "Bird Genius," "Dogs & Super Senses," and "Who's the Smartest?" They aired on PBS April 9, 16, and 23, 2014. The NOVA program can be accessed through http://video.pbs.org/video/2365222887/ or http://www.pbs.org/wgbh/nova/nature/inside-animal-minds.html#animal-minds-dogs.

A related NOVA scienceNOW transcript of a Q&A session with the leader of the Dog Cognition Lab in New York City, Dr. Alexandra Horowitz, also discusses John Pilley and Chaser: http://www.pbs.org/wgbh/nova/nature/horowitz-dogs.html.

6 Information provided by the UC Berkeley Newscenter, September, 2014.
7 In her column, Dr. Gourguechon concludes her essay as follows:

> Dr. Hobson goes on to report that he has found that "dreaming is a parallel state of consciousness that is continually running but normally suppressed during waking." Wait a minute. Isn't this a perfect description of the *unconscious*? Maybe even neurophysiological evidence for the existence of the unconscious?
>
> In my clinical work, I relate to dreams as stories a patient constructs using images, plays on words, narrative twists, juxtapositions, and emotional saturation to communicate to himself and to me something that cannot yet be told in ordinary ways. Actually, this fits with Dr. Hobson's idea that "dreams are tuning the mind for conscious awareness." But he seems to be referring to the mind at its most mundane level (just being awake) while I see a dream as a way of preparing the mind for awareness at the very highest levels of complex meanings, painful feelings, new possibilities. I am always struck by how much more creative we can be in our dreams than in our waking life.

From "The Meaning of Dreams and Do Dreams have Meaning," by Prudence Gourguechon, M.D. in *Psychology Today*, November 10, 2009. Accessed through: http://www.psychologytoday.com/blog/psychoanalytic-excavation/200911/the-meaning-dreams-and-do-dreams-have-meaning.

8 Sonu Shamdasani's *Introduction* to *Liber Novus: The "Red Book" of C. G. Jung* provides valuable background – partly biographical and historical and in part contextual – for Jung's dreams and images. For instance, the following paragraphs describe his interest in spiritualism, trances, and seances:

> The latter half of the nineteenth century witnessed the emergence of modern spiritualism, which spread across Europe and America. Through spiritualism, the cultivation of trances – with the attendant phenomena of trance speech, glossolalia, automatic writing, and crystal vision – became widespread. The phenomena of spiritualism attracted the interest of leading scientists such as Crookes, Zollner, and Wallace. It also attracted the interest of psychologists, including Freud, Ferenczi, James Janet, Stanley Hall and many others.
>
> (Shamdasani 2009, 195)

> During his university days in Basel, Jung and his fellow students took part in séances. In 1896, they engaged in a long series of sittings with his cousin Helene Preiswerk, who appeared to have mediumistic abilities. Jung found that during the trances, she would become different personalities, and that he could call up these personalities by suggestion.
>
> (Shamdasani 2009, 195)

Jung's medical dissertation focused on the psychogenesis of spiritual-
istic phenomena, in the form of an analyses of his séances with Helene
Preiswerk.

(Shamdasani 2009, 195)

9 The 55th Venice Biennale was held from June 1 to November 24, 2014,
and included the works of 185 artists from 88 countries. The exhibit was
curated by Massimiliano Gioni, the New York City-based art critic. In an
essay included in the first volume of the Biennale's catalog ("Is Everything
in My Mind?"), he explained some of the motivating thoughts that were the
leitmotif for Biennale and the choice of works. Also, the connection with this
year's exhibit and our minds, dreams, hallucinations, and visions:

What room is left for internal images – for dreams, hallucinations and
visions – in an era besieged by external ones? And what is the point of
creating an image of the world when the world itself has become increasingly like an image?

. . .

We are not the only animals that carry images embedded in our minds and
bodies, but as humans we are the only animals that create and give life to
images. "The human being is the natural locus of images, a living organ for
images," writes Hans Belting. [Note: quotation from Hans Belting. 2011.
An Anthropology of Images. Princeton, NJ: Princeton University Press.)].
The observation that our minds and bodies are equally inhabited by, and
the source of, our images is a truism as profound as it is disarming in its
simplicity. The experience of art may well owe its power to the paradox
of perceiving external, artificial images that appear to be manifestations of
our inner ones. It is here, in this encounter between internal and external
images, that the sense of a small miracle resides.

. . .

Nowhere are we more justified in speaking of ourselves as "the locus of
images" than when it comes to dreams.

The quotes above are from *Is Everything in My Mind?* by Massimiliano Gioni,
Curator and Director, 55th International Art Exhibition (Fondazione La Biennale
di Venezia), pages 23 to 28 of *Il Palazzo Enciclopedico*, Volume I, Catalogue
of *Biennale Arte 2013, la Biennale di Venezia, 55. Esposizione Internazionale
d'Arte.* 2013. Venice: Marsilio Editori.

10 Mihaly Csikszentmihalyi was born in Fiume, Italy (now Rijeka, Croatia) in
1934. He emigrated to the United States from Hungary at the age of 22 and
is now at Claremont Graduate University. He earned his B.A. (1960) and his
Ph.D. (1965) at the University of Chicago, where he returned in 1969 as a professor and became chair of the Department of Psychology. Csikszentmihalyi is
best known for his theory of flow, which he outlined in his seminal 1990 book
Flow: The Psychology of Optimal Experience. According to Csikszentmihalyi,
people are happy when they are in a state of flow, a type of intrinsic motivation that involves being fully focused on the situation or task.

In a TED talk delivered in February, 2004, he summarized his theory.
The paragraphs quoted below are from the transcript that is available in
30 languages and can be accessed through: http://www.ted.com/talks/mihaly_
csikszentmihalyi_on_flow?language=en and http://www.ted.com/talks/mihaly_
csikszentmihalyi_on_flow/transcript?language=en.

0:11 I grew up in Europe, and World War II caught me when I was between seven and ten years old. And I realized how few of the grown-ups that I knew were able to withstand the tragedies that the war visited on them – how few of them could even resemble a normal, contented, satisfied, happy life once their job, their home, their security was destroyed by the war. So I became interested in understanding what contributed to a life that was worth living.

13:56 Now, when we do studies – we have, with other colleagues around the world, done over 8,000 interviews of people – from Dominican monks, to blind nuns, to Himalayan climbers, to Navajo shepherds – who enjoy their work. And regardless of the culture, regardless of education or whatever, there are these seven conditions that seem to be there when a person is in flow. There's this focus that, once it becomes intense, leads to a sense of ecstasy, a sense of clarity: you know exactly what you want to do from one moment to the other; you get immediate feedback. You know that what you need to do is possible to do, even though difficult, and sense of time disappears, you forget yourself, you feel part of something larger. And once the conditions are present, what you are doing becomes worth doing for its own sake.

11 From the Positive Psychology Center's website, University of Pennsylvania, Philadelphia (http://www.positivepsychology.org/index.html):

> *Dr. Martin E.P. Seligman* is the Director of the Center and a Professor of Psychology. He is a leading authority in the fields of Positive Psychology, resilience, learned helplessness, depression, optimism and pessimism. He is also an expert on interventions that prevent depression, and build strengths and well-being. He has written more than 250 scholarly publications and about 20 books, including "Authentic Happiness" (2002, New York: Simon & Schuster / Atria) and "Learned Optimism" (Vintage Edition, 2005).
>
> *Positive Psychology* is the scientific study of the strengths and virtues that enable individuals and communities to thrive. The field is founded on the belief that people want to lead meaningful and fulfilling lives, to cultivate what is best within themselves, and to enhance their experiences of love, work, and play.

12 http://www.ted.com/talks/martin_seligman_on_the_state_of_psychology? language=en
   So far the video talk apparently has been viewed almost three million times (and it exists with subtitles in 31 languages). The transcript (from which I just copied the first two or so minutes) is available in 29 languages.

13 Transcript of the first two minutes of Dr. Seligman's TED Talk (2008)
   http://www.ted.com/talks/martin_seligman_on_the_state_of_psychology/ transcript?language=en

> 0:11 When I was president of the American Psychological Association, they tried to media-train me, and an encounter I had with CNN summarizes what I'm going to be talking about today, which is the 11th reason to be optimistic. The editor of Discover told us ten of them, I'm going to give you the 11th.
>
> 0:35 So they came to me – CNN – and they said, "Professor Seligman, would you tell us about the state of psychology today? We'd like to interview you about that." And I said, "Great." And she said, "But this is CNN, so you only get a sound bite." So I said, "Well, how many words do I get?" And she said, "Well, one."
>
> 0:57 (Laughter)

0:58 And cameras rolled, and she said, "Professor Seligman, what is the state of psychology today?" "Good."

1:08 (Laughter)

1:10 "Cut. Cut. That won't do. We'd really better give you a longer sound bite." "Well, how many words do I get this time?" "I think, well, you get two. Doctor Seligman, what is the state of psychology today?" "Not good."

1:29 (Laughter)

1:38 "Look, Doctor Seligman, we can see you're really not comfortable in this medium. We'd better give you a real sound bite. This time you can have three words. Professor Seligman, what is the state of psychology today?" "Not good enough." And that's what I'm going to be talking about.

1:59 I want to say why psychology was good, why it was not good and how it may become, in the next ten years, good enough. And by parallel summary, I want to say the same thing about technology, about entertainment and design, because I think the issues are very similar.

2:16 So, why was psychology good? Well, for more than 60 years, psychology worked within the disease model. Ten years ago, when I was on an airplane and I introduced myself to my seatmate, and told them what I did, they'd move away from me. And because, quite rightly, they were saying psychology is about finding what's wrong with you. Spot the loony. And now, when I tell people what I do, they move toward me.

References

Barabasz, Arreed and John G. Watkins. 2005. *Hypnotherapeutic Techniques,* 2nd ed. New York: Brunner-Rutledge.

Barnett, Edgar A. and John R. Tkach. 2005. *The Rapid Reintegration Procedure. Effective Ego State Hypnotherapy Without Hypnosis.* Ontario: Junica.

Csikszentmihalyi, M. 1990. *Flow: The Psychology of Optimal Experience.* New York: HarperCollins.

Gioni, Massimiliano. 2013. *Is Everything in My Mind?* In Volume I, Catalogue of *Biennale Arte 2013, la Biennale di Venezia, 55. Esposizione Internazionale d'Arte.* Fondazione La Biennale di Venezia. Venice: Marsilio Editori, pp. 23–28.

Hobson, J. Allan. 1988. *The Dreaming Brain: How the Brain Creates Both the Sense and Nonsense of Dreams.* New York: Basic Books.

Hobson, J. Allan. 2001. *The Dream Drugstore: Chemically Altered States of Consciousness.* Cambridge: MIT Press.

Hobson, J. Allan. 2002. *Dreaming: An Introduction to the Science of Sleep.* Oxford: Oxford University Press.

Hobson, J. Allan and Hellmut Wohl. 2005. *From Angels to Neurones: Art and the New Science of Dreaming.* Special Edition. Mattioli 1885.

Jung, C. G. 1989. *Memories, Dreams, Reflections.* Revised ed. Recorded by Aniela Jaffe. Translated by Richard and Clara Winston. New York: Vintage Books.

Jung, C. G. 2009. *The Red Book (Liber Novus).* Edited by Sonu Shamdasani; translated by Mark Kyburz, John Peck, and Sonu Shamdasani (Philemon Series). New York: W. W. Norton.

Kaku, M. 2014. *The Future of the Mind: The Scientific Quest to Understand, Enhance, and Empower the Mind.* New York: Doubleday.

Kim, Meeri. 2013. "Brains Flush Toxic Waste in Sleep, Including Alzheimer's-Linked Protein, Study of Mice Finds." *The Washington Post*, October 19.

Kurzweil, R. 2012. *How to Create A Mind: The Secret of Human Thought Revealed*. New York: The Penguin Group.

Lynn, Steven J. and Judith W. Rhue. 1991. *Theories of Hypnosis: Current Models and Perspectives*. New York. Guilford Press.

Rossi, E. and K. Rossi. 2006. "The Neuroscience of Observing Conscious and Mirror Neurons in Therapeutic Hypnosis." *American Journal of Clinical Hypnosis* 48: 278–283.

Shamdasani, Sonu, editor. 2009. Introduction. *Liber Novus: The "Red Book" of C.G. Jung*. Translated by Mark Kyburz, John Peck, and Sonu Shamdasani. New York: W. W. Norton, pp. 194–221.

Underwood, Emily. 2013. "Sleep: The Brain's Housekeeper?" *Science* 342 (18 October): 301.

von Neumann, J. 2012.. *The Computer and the Brain*, 3rd ed. New Haven, Conn.: Yale University Press. (Foreword by Ray Kurzweil.)

Xie, Lulu, Hongyi Kang, Qiwu Xu, Michael J. Chen, Yonghong Liao, Meenakshisundaram Thiyagarajan, John O'Donnell, Daniel J. Christensen, Charles Nicholson, Jeffrey J. Iliff, Takahiro Takano, Rashid Deane, Maiken Nedergaard. 2013. "Sleep Drives Metabolite Clearance from the Adult Brain." *Science* 342 (6156): 373–377.

Zimmer, C. 2014 "Secrets of the Brain." *National Geographic* 225 (2): 28–57.

Appendix A

Sleep patterns in 2-year-old children

William C. Kohler, A.B., R. Dean Coddington, M.D., and H. W. Agnew, Jr., M.A.

GAINESVILLE, FLA.

Sleep disturbances in children tend to be diagnosed and treated on an empirical basis. Methods are now available for more objective treatment of these disturbances. The sleep patterns of 16 healthy 2-year-old children were analyzed with all night electroencephalography and electrooculography. The characteristic sleep patterns of this age group and the possible use of this information in clinical medicine are discussed. The relationship between sleep and dream patterns and chronological and mental age, as well as dreaming, in this age group is reported.

THE DETECTION, diagnosis, and treatment of sleep problems in the infant are classically handled in an empirical fashion based on the pediatrician's clinical experience, but rarely from a neurophysiological point of view. Recent widespread use of all night electroencephalography and electrooculography in the study of both normal and disturbed sleep in adults and adolescents presents the pediatrician and child psychiatrist with a new tool for the study of the sleep of children. This technique has revealed that there are some aspects of sleep which are typical of an individual and others which are typical of the sleep of all subjects studied.[1,2] For example, individuals have been observed to spend a characteristic amount of time in each stage of sleep night after night. Within

narrow age limits, however, there is a typical sleep pattern for a group of subjects. Studies of the normative characteristics of sleep at the University of Florida have been done in the following age groups: 30 to 40, 50 to 60, and 60 to 70 years. However, few normative studies are available on the sleep characteristics of subjects below the age of 8 years. Onheiber and associates,[3] Parmelee and colleagues,[4] and Roffwarg, Dement, and Fisher[5] are currently working with young children, but have thus far reported their results for only a few subjects.

Particular attention has been focused on the characteristics of 2 of the electroencephalographic stages of sleep. In 1955, Aserinsky and Kleitman[6] observed an association of rapid eye movements with the low voltage fast activity seen in the electroencephalogram of patients in "stage 1 sleep." When subjects were awakened from this stage 1, rapid—eye-movement, phase of sleep, a high incidence of dream recall was observed. Furthermore, Dement[7] observed 2 main responses in subjects deprived of rapid—eye-movement sleep. First, with continued deprivation there were more intrusions of rapid—eye-movement sleep into the individual's pattern. Second, on un-disturbed nights following such deprivation subjects showed a marked preference for rapid—eye-movement sleep.

Stage 4 sleep has also received considerable attention. This type of sleep is characterized by a high amplitude (200 to 400 microvolts) slow waves (0.5 to 3 c.p.s.) in the electroencephalograph. When Agnew, Webb, and Williams[8] deprived subjects of this stage of sleep, there were increased intrusions of slow waves in the individual's sleep pattern, and on undisturbed nights following such deprivation subjects showed a marked preference for stage 4 sleep. Furthermore, when subjects deprived of stage 4 sleep were given psychometric tests, their profiles indicated that the deprivation produced a depressive and hypochondriacal reaction.

Recent work in our laboratory with a pair of 23-month-old identical twins, one of whom was developmentally retarded, revealed that the sleep pattern may indicate the stage of development of the infant's central nervous system. The developmentally retarded twin showed a consistently greater amount of rapid—eye-movement than her normal sister. As the retarded infant's psychological development improved, the percent of rapid—eye-movement sleep decreased toward the value of her normal sister's. This suggested the possible use of the sleep electroencephalograph in detecting developmental retardation. Insufficient normative data for 2-year-old infants were present in the literature, however, for such an investigation.

The present study is an attempt to help meet the need for normative data on the very young, and specifically to answer the following questions: (1) Is the sleep pattern of the 2-year-old child significantly different from that of the young adult? (2) What is the typical amount of time that the 2-year-old child spends in stages 4 and rapid—eye-movement sleep? (3) Is there a correlation between mental age or chronological age and either stage 4 or rapid—eye-movement sleep? (4) Does dreaming occur during rapid—eye-movement sleep in the very young as it does in the adult?

Subjects and Methods

Sixteen healthy 2-year-old children, 8 male and 8 female, were studied. Their ages ranged from 21 to 31 months (mean, 25.7). The subjects were drawn from the families of university students and employees. Physical examinations were performed on all subjects and only those found to be free of organic disease were used. The Stanford-Binet test, form L-M, was administered to each subject within a week of his electroencephalograph recordings by a psychologist who had no knowledge of the subject's sleep pattern.

The subjects were brought to the laboratory 1 hour earlier than their usual bedtime to be wired for the electroencephalograph and electrooculograph. The International Ten-Twenty system was used to locate electrode sites for recording a 6 channel electroencephalograph between F_1-C_5, F_2-C_6, C_1-C_5, C_2-C_6, C_1-o_1, C_2-o_2 In addition, sites were located about the eyes for recording a 4 channel electrooculograph trace between the inferior canthus of the left eye and the superior canthus of the right eye, inferior canthus of the left **eye** and F_1, superior canthus of the right eye and nasion, and inferior canthus of the left eye and nasion. The electroencephalograph machines were run continuously throughout the night at a paper speed of 15 mm. per second. An experimenter was in constant attendance. Four consecutive nights were recorded on each subject; however, only the last 3 nights are reported here.

The records were scored with a modification of the Dement and Kleitman[9] (1957) system. Each record was scored by a well-trained scorer and cross checked by an independent scorer to achieve a reliability of 90 per cent. Each 9 to 10 hour record was divided into 1 minute epochs and scored, minute by minute, with the following criteria*:

Stage 0   Epoch composed of atleast 30 seconds of 8 to 12 c.p.s occipital activity. This stage corresponds to the waking state.

Stage 1   Epoch composed of less than 30 seconds of 8 to 12 c.p.s. activity and no more than 1 spindle or K complex.

Stage 2   Epoch composed of 2 spindles or 2 K complexes or 1 of each, and no more than 20 seconds of slow waves (1 to 3 c.p.s.)

Stage 4   Epoch composed of more than 20 seconds of delta (1 to 3 c.p.s.)

Stage 1-REM   A stage 1 electroencephalogram plus evidence of rapid eye movements. This is the dream phase of sleep.

In an attempt to determine whether or not dreams occur in 2-year-old children, 6 subjects, chosen because of their verbal abilities, were asked to return to the sleep laboratory for a fifth night. The mothers of 4 of the subjects also slept in the laboratory. The children were awakened a total of 35 times randomly throughout the night. They were asked to describe such things as what they had been doing, what they had seen, and whom they were with. In some cases the mother was awakened and she interrogated them.

In this study, dreams were defined as any verbal production that was out of context with the experimental situation. The definition was narrowed in this manner as to avoid misconstruing statements made while awake as dream material. Such description as those of playmates, certain activities outside of the laboratory, animals, and television were considered to be representative of dreams.

Tape recordings were made of all attempts to awaken the children and were reviewed by a child psychiatrist (R. Dean Coddington), who had no knowledge of the presence or absence of rapid—eye-movement periods preceding the awakening. Each awakening was then scored as to the presence or absence of dream material. Finally, reference was made to the existence of rapid eye movement preceding the awakenings, and the findings were correlated.

Results

The length of the sleep records ranged from 506 to 683 minutes, with an average of 597 minutes. In Table I is recorded the mean per cent of total sleep each subject spent in each stage of sleep. Two features of these data should be noted. First, there is a wide range of individual differences in the time spent in each stage of sleep. It can be seen that this range for rapid—eye-movement sleep is from 17.9 to 36.4 per cent (mean, 28.7 per cent); and

for stage 4, from 13.4 to 22.9 per cent (mean, 17.6 per cent). Second, although there are large individual differences in these data, the relatively small values obtained for the standard deviations of these measures indicate a tendency for most of the scores to be grouped about the mean, making it possible to utilize the means at the bottom of the table as the typical sleep pattern for subjects of this age.

The sleep of these subjects was also examined in terms of the number of shifts from one stage to another which occurred during the night. When this variable was examined, it was found that this group of subjects produced an average of 3.5 shifts per hour slept. A detailed examination of the rapid—eye-movement periods revealed that there was an average of 7.6 rapid—eye movement periods per night with a mean length of 22.6 minutes each.

The characteristics of the sleep stages in each third of the sleep period are seen in Table II. This analysis shows that 66.2 per cent of the total stage 4 sleep time occurred during the first third of the sleep period, while only 8.5 per cent of the total stage 4 sleep occurred during the last part of the sleep period. On the other hand, relatively little of the rapid—eye-movement sleep occurred during the first third of sleep, while 48.2 per cent of this type of sleep appeared during the last third of sleep.

The sequence in which one stage follows another is a third characteristic of sleep. To obtain this measure a contingency table

Table I Mean Per cent of total sleep time for five stages of sleep taken during the consecutive nights for each subject

Subject	Sleep stage				
	0*	1	Rem†	2	4
1	0.9	7.9	27.4	44.7	19.0
2	0.0	3.5	32.0	47.8	16.7
3	0.3	7.7	32.7	44.8	14.4
4	8.4	8.6	21.2	42.0	19.8
5	1.7	11.9	17.9	51.1	17.3
6	1.0	6.2	25.4	50.0	17.4
7	5.0	7.6	35.0	35.0	17.2
8	1.6	4.7	31.6	46.8	15.3
9	0.2	6.8	33.5	38.8	20.7
10	2.7	7.3	28.8	47.8	13.4
11	2.4	11.2	28.4	41.2	16.8
12	1.1	7.1	26.2	42.8	22.9
13	1.2	10.9	25.6	41.2	21.1
14	0.4	6.8	36.4	39.4	17.0
15	2.1	8.7	22.9	47.4	19.0
16	2.9	7.6	34.4	40.6	14.5
Mean %	1.9	7.7	28.7	43.8	17.6
Mean minutes	11.9	46.5	171.3	261.6	105.3
Standard deviation	2.1	2.2	5.3	4.5	2.6

* Time awake after onset of sleep.

†REM = rapid eye movement.

Table II Percentage of time spent in each sleep stage during each third of the night

Sleep Stage	Thirds		
	I	II	III
0	18.1	33.0	48.9
1	38.5	37.2	24.3
REM*	16.4	35.4	48.2
2	30.7	34.5	34.7
4	66.2	25.3	8.5

* REM = rapid eye movement.

was constructed and the number of times a particular stage of sleep was followed by the other stages was tallied. The resulting percentages are given in Table **III**. It can be seen from this table that the sleep of these subjects was very smooth, involving a progression of only one stage at a time, both when sleep was deepening and lightening.

The Pearson product moment correlation was used to determine if

Table III Sequence of sleep stage changes in terms of per cent of time one stage was followed by another

Following stage	This sleep stage			
	0	1	2	4
0	–	7.3	4.6	1.6
1	97.8	–	53.6	6.4
2	2.2	92.7	–	92.0
4	0.0	0.0	41.8	–

there was a relationship between 2 of the sleep stages (4 and rapid eye movement) and 2 measures of age (chronological and mental). These correlations are shown in Table IV. The intelligence quotients (I.Q.'s) ranged from 59 to 130. When a t test was used to test the significance of these correlations, it was found that the −0.41 correlation between mental age and the per cent of stage rapid-eyemovement sleep and the −0.37 correlation between chronological age and the per cent of stage 4 sleep were not significant at the 0.05 level.

The results of random awakenings during the night in an attempt to obtain dream recall are shown in Table V. We were unable to get any verbal descriptions from three children, regardless of whether

Table IV Correlation matrix for chronological age and mental age and stages 4 and REM*

Chronological age		Mental age
REM	−0.21	−0.41
4	−0.37	−0.11

* REM = rapid eye movement.

Table V Dream recall during random awakening

Subject No.	REM* awakenings		Non-REM awakenings	
	No.	Dream recall (%)	NO.	Dream recall (%)
2	3	66	1	0
8	3	100	4	0
10	4	0	3	0
12	5	0	2	0
13	3	0	4	0
15	2	50	1	0
Total	20	30	15	0

* REM = rapid eyemovement.

they were awakened from rapid eye movement or non-rapid eye movement. Three children consistently reported dream material when awakened during rapid eye movement, and none reported dream material when awakened during nonrapid—eye-movement periods. The total results were 30 per cent dream recall when awakened during rapid eye movement and 0 per cent when awakened during non-rapid eye movement. These findings suggest that 2-year-old children do dream during the night and that rapid—eyemovement sleep is associated with dream recall.

Discussion

The findings of this study represent an attempt to better define the normative sleep pattern of 2-year-old children. These results, along with the work of authors such as Parmelee[4] and Roffwarg[5] and their associates, give a clearer understanding of the basic sleep characteristics which are unique to this age group.

The percentage of time spent in each stage of sleep in this group of subjects can he compared with various other age groups. Two-year-old children obtain a greater percentage of rapid—eye-movement sleep than do older subjects who have been studied in this laboratory.[1] It also appears that the 2-year-old child spends more time in stage 4. Due to the assignment of time spent in stage 3 into stages 2 or 4, however, a valid comparison between stage 4 in 2-year-old children and in other age groups cannot be made.

The relatively small number of sleep stage changes was one of the striking features of sleep in the infant. The 3.5 stage shifts per hour were significantly different from the 5.3 stage shifts observed in young adults. Another unique characteristic of sleep in this age group was the smooth progression of stages whether moving toward stage 4 or stage 0. In contrast, when the sleep of the young adults was lightening, it frequently involved a jump of more than one stage.

It is also of interest that we were able to elicit dream responses during rapid—eyemovement sleep in this age group. This finding is in agreement with that of Dement and Kleitman,[10] who found that in adults the majority of dreaming occurs during rapid—eye-movement sleep.

While our work does not show a significant relationship between mental age and rapid—eye-movement sleep, it does indicate such a trend, and further work in this area is definitely warranted, The establishment of a relationship between the sleep pattern and the developmental age of a child would be of significant value in diagnostic and therapeutic work with retarded and emotionally disturbed children. Our results should serve as useful normative data for further exploration.

Summary

The sleep patterns of 16 two-year-old subjects are described. Although there are considerable individual differences, it is possible to utilize the mean sleep stage values as the typical sleep pattern for this age group. Characteristically, most of rapid—eye-movement sleep occurs in the *last* third of the night, whereas most of stage 4 sleep occurs in the *first* third. The 2-year-old child spends approximately 29 per cent of the night in rapid—eye-movement sleep. Changes in sleep stage are relatively infrequent, and when they do occur the progression is smooth.

The relationship between sleep stage (1—rapid eye movement and 4) and age (chronological and mental) was investigated. The trend was a negative correlation between rapid—eye-movement sleep per cent and chronological and mental age. Further work is indicated.

Dreaming in this age group was also investigated. Dream responses were elicited after awakenings from rapid—eye-movement sleep but not after awakenings from nonrapid—eye-movement periods.

The authors wish to acknowledge the assistance of Mary Francis Robertson, M.A., who administered and scored the psychological tests

Note

* The scoring of stage 3 was found to be unreliable in this age group. What would have normally been stage 3 was distributed into stages 2 and 4.

References

1 Williams, R. L., Agnew, Jr., H. W., and Webb, W. B.: Sleep patterns in young adults: An EEG study. Electroencephalog. & Clin. Neurophysiol. 17: 376, 1964.

2 Williams, R. L., Agnew, Jr., H. W., and Webb, W. B.: Sleep patterns in the young adult female: An EEG study. Electroencephalog. & Clin. Neurophysiol. 20: 264, 1966.

3 Onheiber, P., White, P. T., DeMyer, M., and Ottinger, D. R.: Sleep and dream patterns of child schizophrenics, Arch. Gen. Psychiat. 12: 568, 1965.

4 Parmelee, A. H., Wenner, W., Akiyama, T., and Flescher, J.: Electroencephalography and brain maturation. *CIOMS* symposium on regional maturation of the nervous system in early life, Paris, December, 1964.

5 Roffwarg, H., Dement, W., and Fisher, C.: Preliminary observation of the sleep-dream pattern in neonates, infants, children, and adults, *in* Hams, E., editor: Problems of sleep and dreams in children, New York, 1964, The Macmillan Company.

6 Aserinsky, E., and Kleitman, N.: Two types of ocular motility occurring in sleep, J. Appl. Physiol. 8; 1, 1955.

7 Dement, W.: The effect of dream deprivation, Science 131: 1705, 1960.

8 Agnew, Jr., H. W., Webb, W. B., and Williams, R. L.: Comparison of stage four and 1-REM sleep deprivation, Perceptual. & Motor Skills 24: 851, 1967.

9 Dement, W., and Kleitman, N.: Cyclic variations in EEG during sleep and their relation to eye movements, body motility, and dreaming, Electroenceph. clin. Neurophysiol. 9: 673, 1957.

10 Dement, W., and Kleitman, N.: The relation of eye movements during sleep to dream activity: An objective method for the study of dreaming, J. Exper. Psychol. 53: 339, 1957.

Appendix B

The Treatment of Sleepwalking with Hypnosis

Kohler, William C.M.D.

FLORIDA SLEEP INSTITUTE, SPRING HILL, FLORIDA

Poster by William C. Kohler, M.D., presented at the 4th International Congress of the World Association of Sleep Medicine (WASM) – 75th Conference of the Canadian Sleep Society (CSS), September 10–14, 2011, Quebec City, Canada. The poster describes and summarizes a research project by Dr. Kohler, conducted at the Florida Sleep Institute, Spring Hill, Florida. It was reproduced in Volume 12, September 2011 (Abstracts, Supplement 1, S1-S138), of *Sleep Medicine*, the official journal of WASM and of the International Pediatric Sleep Association (www. sleep-journal.com)

Introduction and Objectives

Hypnosis has been successfully applied in treating parasomnias including sleepwalking, nightmares, night terrors and sleep related eating disorders. (1) (2) (3) Hypnosis with a unique post hypnotic suggestion was utilized successfully in treating sleepwalking in a sleep medicine practice.

Acknowledgements

(1) Hauri, PJ, Silber. MH, Boeve, BF. The Treatment of Parasomnia with Hypnosis: A 5 Year Follow-Up Study *J. Clin Sleep Med.* 2007; 3(4): 369-73.
(2) Hurwitz, TD. Mahowald, MW. Schenck, CH. Schluter, JL. Bundie, SR. A retrospective outcome study and review of hypnosis as treatment of adults with sleepwalking and sleep terror *J. Nerv Ment Dis.* 1991; 179.
(3) Reid, WH. Ahmed, I. Levie, CA. Treatment of Sleepwalking: A controlled study. *Am. J. Pschother* 1981; 35:27-37. 228-233.

Materials and methods

Twelve patients seen for treatment of sleepwalking were treated with hypnosis. Hypnotherapy was performed by the author who is a board certified sleep specialist and an Approved Consultant in Clinical Hypnosis by the American Society of Clinical Hypnosis. Hypnosis was performed using visual imagery induction with images chosen by the patient prior to the hypnotherapy. The patient was seated with his feet on a stool. Post hypnotic suggestions included ego strengthening and the suggestion that "whenever your feet touch the floor you will immediately be awake and will go back to sleep as soon as you want to". Following the initial session, the patient was asked to evaluate how he felt and to suggest changes in the wording of the post-hypnotic suggestion. A second session was held immediately thereafter and a tape was made. The patients were asked to practice the tape at least once a day.

Results

Twelve patients, 6 females and 6 males, underwent hypnotherapy. Their ages ranged from 11½ years to 77 years, with onset of sleepwalking ranging from preschool to age 64 (see Table 1). The number of sessions ranged from 1 to 3. At the time of the initial evaluation, all 12 patients showed cessation or marked reduction in sleepwalking. Eight patients who were followed from between 3 and 42 months reported complete cessation in sleepwalking (see Table 2).

Table 1

Patient	Age (yrs)	Sex	Age at Onset (yrs)	Frequency of events (per month)
1	52	F	age 51	8
2	54	F	childhood	4
3	12 3/12	M	age 12	3
4	11 6/12	M	age 10	90
5	50	M	age 49	60
6	16	M	age 15	varies
7	27	F	preschool	<1
8	77	F	age 64	12
9	12 6/12	M	age 12	30
10	54	F	age 53	4
11	29	M	age 9	1, varies
12	16	F	age 16	30

Table 2

Patient	# hypnosis sessions	Short-term improvement		Long-term improvement	
		(# episodes)	*(period)*	*(# episodes)*	*(period)*
1	1	0	8 weeks	0	8 months
2	1	0	12 days	0	33 months
3	1	0	2 weeks	0	2 months
4	1			"doing very well"	12 months
5	2	0	2 months		
6	3	rare, improved	3 months	0	42 months
7	1	rare, improved	6 weeks	0	3 months
8	1	0	3 weeks		
9	1	improved	3 months	0	6 months
10	1	0	1 month	0	3 months
11	1	0	2 weeks		
12	1			markedly improvement	10 months

Conclusion

Hypnotherapy is an effective and safe treatment for sleepwalking.

Appendix C
Glossary

Abreaction The experience and discharge of emotion concerning a psychological condition. During hypnosis the patient may abreact the emotion of previously expressed conflicts.

Active sleep A term used for the sleep state in the neonate which is considered equivalent to REM (rapid eye movement) sleep.

Age regression By suggestion, the patient is caused to revert to an earlier age.

Alpha activity An alpha EEG wave or sequence of waves with a frequency of 8–13 Hz.

Alpha rhythm An EEG rhythm with a frequency of 8–13 Hz. This rhythm is most prominent over the occipital cortex. Alpha rhythm is present during relaxed wakefulness when the eyes are closed.

Amnesia By suggestion, certain items are blocked temporarily from memory (this is known as partial amnesia). Total amnesia may be produced for a certain period of time.

Arm levitation A technique used in hypnosis in which the arm is made to feel light by suggestion and lifts up into the air.

Arousal An abrupt change in sleep from a "deeper" stage of NREM to a "lighter" one or from REM toward wakefulness with the possibility of awakening which may be accompanied by increased tonic activity, heart rate, and body movement.

Autohypnosis (self-hypnosis) The act of hypnotizing one's self.

Beta activity An EEG wave or sequence of waves with a frequency of 14–30 Hz.

Beta rhythm An EEG rhythm of 14–30 Hz. The beta rhythm may be associated with alert wakefulness or vigilance and is accompanied by a high tonic electromyogram.

Bruxism Tooth grinding or tooth clenching.

Catalepsy A state of muscular rigidity usually with the antagonistic muscles simultaneously contracted. Catalepsy may be of the whole body or a portion of it.

Cataplexy Sudden decrease in muscle tone and loss of deep tendon reflexes leading to muscle weakness, or paralysis. It is usually triggered by laughter, anger, surprise, or other emotional stimuli. It is one symptom of the narcoleptic tetrad.

Catecholamine　A chemical which acts as a neurotransmitter in the central nervous system such as dopamine, epinephrine, and norepinephrine.

Circadian　About a day or 24 hours, from the Latin *circa* (about) and *diem* (day).

Circadian rhythm　An innate daily fluctuation of function, including sleep–wake states generally tied to a 24-hour cycle.

Cycle　Characteristic of an event which exhibits rhythmic fluctuations. One cycle is defined as the activity from one maximum or minimum to the next.

Declarative memory　Memory which is consciously recalled and can be expressed in words.

Deepening methods　Methods which are designed to help a subject go into a deeper level of hypnosis.

Dehypnotizing　Helping the patient to come out of a hypnotic trance.

Delta activity　EEG activity with a frequency of less that 4 Hz (usually 0.1–3.5 Hz). For sleep staging, delta activity must be 0.5–2 Hz with an amplitude greater than 75 µV, measured over the frontal regions.

Delta sleep stage　Stage of sleep in which EEG delta waves are prevalent or predominant; stage N3, slow-wave sleep.

Dissociation　A splitting of one part of the personality from another. This may be produced in some patients by hypnotic suggestions.

EEG power　The quantity of select frequency bands in the EEG.

Ego strengthening　Suggestions used during hypnosis to increase self-esteem and self-worth.

Electroencephalogram (EEG)　Recording the electrical activity of the brain by means of electrodes placed on the surface of the scalp.

Electromyogram (EMG)　A recording of the muscles by means of electrodes placed over muscle groups. The three basic variables used to score sleep stages and wakefulness are the chin EMG, the EEG and the EOG.

Electro-oculogram (EOG)　A recording of voltage changes resulting from shifts in the position of the eyes. The eyes have a positive (anterior) and negative (posterior) dipole.

Entrainment　Synchronization of a biologic rhythm by a forcing stimulus such as light (*Zeitgeber*).

Enuresis　Inability to control urination. When it occurs during sleep it is known as nocturnal enuresis or bedwetting.

Epworth Sleepinesss Scale (ESS)　An eight-item questionnaire which gives a subjective estimate of sleepiness.

Excessive daytime sleepiness (EDS)　A patient complaint of abnormally high need to sleep, lack of alertness with difficulty maintaining wakefulness during the waking hours.

Finger levitation   The lifting of a finger in an involuntary manner – the patient knows that the finger is lifting but does not feel that s/he is lifting it.

Gamma activity   An EEG wave or sequence of waves with a frequency of 30–50 Hz, centered on 40 Hz.

Hallucination   Perception that appears real, but does not exist outside the mind. It may be visual, auditory, tactile, or gustatory.

Hand levitation   The lifting of the hand in an involuntary manner.

Hertz (Hz)   The unit of frequency. This term is preferred to cycles per second (cps).

Hypersomnolence   Prolonged sleepiness.

Hypnagogic   Occurrence of an event during the transition from wakefulness to sleep.

Hypnagogic imagery (hallucinations)   Vivid sensory images which occur at sleep onset but are particularly vivid with sleep-onset REM periods. Hypnogogic imagery is a feature of narcolepsy, in which REM periods occur at sleep onset. One of the symptoms of the narcolepsy tetrad but also experienced by some patients who do not have narcolepsy.

Hypnoanalysis   Psychoanalysis carried out with the aid of hypnosis. The patient may show less inhibition under hypnosis, hastening the psychoanalytical process.

Hypnoanesthesia   The blocking of sensation by suggestion. Hypnoanesthesia refers to the blocking of pain and should properly be termed hypnoanalgesia.

Hypnopompic   Occurrence of an event during the transition from sleep to wakefulness at the termination of a sleep episode.

Hypnotic suggestion   A suggestion given while the subject is in the hypnotic state. It is offered to the patient for uncritical acceptance.

Hypnotist   One who helps another enter the hypnotic state.

Hypnotizability   The ability of the patient to go into the hypnotic state or trance.

Indirect suggestion   An idea presented in such a way that the patient does not realize that it is addressed to him or her. Such a suggestion is likely to bring out less resistance.

Insomnia   Difficulty in initiating or maintaining sleep or non-restorative sleep.

K-complex   A sharp, biphasic EEG wave. The initial high-voltage wave goes up (negative) followed by a slower (positive) downward deflection. K-complexes occur spontaneously during NREM sleep and begin and define stage N2 sleep. They are thought to be evoked responses to internal stimuli and have a duration of about 0.5 second. External stimuli may also elicit a K-complex.

Levels of hypnosis   Different depths of hypnosis are recognized depending on the type of suggestion the subject will readily accept.

Levitation   The involuntary raising of a part of the body as a result of hypnotic suggestion.

Mind-set   An attitude or opinion about a topic.

Negative suggestion   A negatively stated suggestion such as "this won't cause pain." Usually negative suggestions are less effective than positive ones.

Neuroplasticity   The ability of the brain to form new neural pathways and adapt as needed.

Nightmare   Term used to denote an unpleasant and/or frightening dream that usually occurs in REM sleep.

Paradoxical sleep   Synonymous with REM sleep, which is the preferred term.

Parasomnia   An experiential or physical phenomenon occurring around the time of sleep. A disorder of arousal, partial arousal, or sleep-stage transition.

Periodic leg movement (PLM)   A rapid partial flexion of the foot at the ankle, extension of the big toe, and partial flexion of the knee and hip that occurs during sleep.

PGO spikes   Ponto-geniculo-occipital spikes. Burst of electrical energy from the pons through the lateral geniculate body to the occipital cortex. These occur during REM and are documented on EEG.

Polysomnogram   The continuous and simultaneous recording of multiple physiologic variables during sleep, including the three basic stage-scoring parameters (EEG, EOG, EMG) and electrocardiogram, respiratory airflow, respiratory movements, leg movements, and other electrophysiologic variables.

Posthypnotic suggestion   A suggestion given during the hypnotic trance which is to be carried out after the termination of the hypnotic state.

Procedural memory   Memory skills which can be performed automatically.

Projection   The attributing of a person's own feelings to someone else.

Quiet sleep   NREM sleep in infants.

Rapid eye movement (REM) sleep   Sleep stage with the highest brain activity, characterized by enhanced brain metabolism, spontaneous rapid eye movements, suppression of resting muscle activity. Hallucinatory dreaming may occur. The EEG shows a relatively low-voltage, mixed-frequency pattern. REM sleep is usually 20–30% of total sleep time in the adult.

Rapport   Harmonious or sympathetic relationship.

Resistance   Some people have difficulty undergoing hypnosis because of erroneous ideas concerning hypnosis or from other causes. Resistance may be conscious (subject to awareness) or unconscious.

Restless-legs syndrome (RLS)   A condition characterized by an uncomfortable sensation in the legs while at rest which may be described as a creeping feeling which is usually relieved to some degree by movement and is more prevalent in the evening or at night. The name was changed to Willis–Ekbom disease. The symptoms may involve other parts of the body than just the legs.

Sleep In hypnosis, this term may be used in induction techniques (as "go deeper asleep"). It is a misnomer because the hypnotic trance is not sleep.

Sleep architecture The NREM–REM sleep-stage and cycle infrastructure of sleep understood from the vantage point of the quantitative relationship of these components to each other.

Sleep cycle The time from the start of NREM sleep to the end of the first REM period. An NREM–REM cycle.

Sleep dept Cumulative effect of sleep loss.

Sleep efficiency The percentage of total sleep time compared to time in bed.

Sleep hygiene The use of behavioral and environmental factors to improve sleep.

Sleep latency The time between "lights out" or bedtime and the onset of sleep.

Sleep log (diary) A daily written record of a person's sleep–wake pattern, including such pertinent information as time of retiring and arising, time in bed, estimated total sleep time, number and duration of sleep interruptions, quality of sleep, daytime naps, use of medication or caffeine, and the nature of activities while awake.

Sleep onset The change from awake to asleep as defined by polysomnographic criteria.

Sleep-onset REM periods (SOREMs) Typically defined as the occurrence of REM sleep within 15 minutes of sleep onset at night or during daytime naps.

Sleep paralysis Immobility of the body which may occur in the transition from sleep to wakefulness or pathologically may occur at sleep onset.

Sleep spindle Spindle-shaped bursts of 11–16 Hz (mainly 12–14 Hz) EEG waveforms that last 0.5–1.5 seconds. The spindle bursts are generally diffuse but are of the highest voltage over the central regions of the head. These waveforms are one of the identifying EEG features of NREM stage N2 sleep. They are generated by the reticular nucleus of the thalamus.

Sleep stage NREM Non-REM sleep, one of the two major sleep stages. It compromises sleep stages N1, N2, and N3.

Sleep stage REM One of the two major sleep stages, characterized by rapid eye movements, low EMG muscle tone, and relatively low mixed-frequency EEG pattern.

Sleep stage N1 (NREM stage N1) Stage N1 sleep is a transitional phase between wakefulness and sleep, which is observed periodically throughout the night, especially following body movement. In the EEG it is characterized by a relatively low-voltage, mixed frequency of 2–7 Hz.

Sleep stage N2 (NREM stage N 2)   A type of NREM sleep defined by the presence of sleep spindles and K-complexes interspersed in a low-voltage 3–7-Hz EEG pattern.

Sleep stage N3 (NREM stage N3)   A type of NREM sleep characterized by 20% or more delta waves.

Slow-wave sleep (SWS)   A type of NREM sleep with a majority of the EEG activity consisting of delta waves (high-amplitude, 0.5–2 Hz).

Suggestibility   A normal characteristic of human beings. The quality of accepting a suggestion. The acceptance of ideas which will modify behavior uncritically and with a minimum of resistance.

Suggestion   An idea so presented to a patient that s/he will accept it with a minimum of analysis, criticism, or resistance which will lead to or modify behavior.

Suprachiasmatic nucleus (SCN)   The anterior region of the hypothalamus identified as a putative pacemaker of circadian rhythm.

Tests of suggestibility   Methods designed to measure the degree of suggestibility of a subject.

Theta rhythm   EEG activity ranging between 4 and 8 Hz.

Trance   Term used to describe the hypnotic experience. The word "state" is also used.

Zeitgeber   An environmental cue to help to entrain or synchronize a physiological activity to a particular cycle. Light is one of the most powerful *Zeitgebers*. A "time-giver."

Appendix D
Resources

During the writing of this book, the authors discussed and envisioned a more ambitious "Resources" section than what the reader will find here. From the beginning Dr. Kohler and I struggled with the conflict between the limited, narrow focus of our work and the much larger field represented by the global nature of the issues related to "sleep" and "hypnosis." Initially we considered selecting relevant quotes for the beginning of each chapter, each one symbolically in a different language. From that we moved to what appeared to be a more practical goal – perhaps more useful to the reader – of assembling a "Resources" appendix that would refer to, include and draw from a large number of academic and research organizations around the world, from those that are somehow connected to the fields of sleep medicine and the use of hypnosis in the management of sleep disorders.

After several phone conversations, we agreed that this would be a valuable addition and planned to create an Appendix that would reflect this global interest and effort. Less than a month before Dr. Kohler's death, the following excerpts from a letter dated September 15, 2014, outlined our joint thinking:

Our works consulted are "mostly from North America, a little bit (from) Europe, and almost (all) exclusively from English language sources. Since we can't possibly cover such an enormous field, the RESOURCES section might help close the gap. If possible, we should go beyond English – especially as it relates to our two key topics.

"(. . .) The most important – the key – topics are SLEEP and HYPNOSIS. Perhaps we could make the RESOURCES section – as it relates to those two key topics – somewhat more global than it now is."

The letter continues by citing numerous centers and publications worldwide where currently there is important research being conducted in these two fields: "(. . .) in addition to AJCH, let's also include American, British, German, French, Spanish, Italian, Russian and 'Other' important journals and associations."

For various reasons, at this time and for this edition, our "Resources" section is limited to the following major and important organizations based in the United States:

American Academy of Sleep Medicine
 2510 North Frontage Road
 Darien IL 60561
 Tel: (630)-737-9700 www.aasmnet.org

American Society of Clinical Hypnosis (ASCH)
 140 Bloomingdale Road
 Bloomingdale IL 60108
 Tel: (630)-980-4740 www.asch.net

National Sleep Foundation
 1010 North Glebe Road, Suite 310
 Arlingon VA 22201
 Tel: (703)-243-1697 www.sleepfoundation.org

Sleep Research Society (SRS)
 2510 North Frontage Road
 Darien IL 60561
 Tel: (630)-787-9702 www.sleepresearchsociety.org

Society for Clinical and Experimental Hypnosis (SCEH)
 305 Commandants Way, Common Cove Suite 100
 Chelsea MA 02150 www.sceh.us

The Milton H. Erickson Foundation
 2632 East Thomas Road, Suite 200
 Phoenix AZ 85016
 Tel: (602)-956-6196 www.erickson-foundation.org

World Sleep Society (WSS)

Founded in 2016 by the World Association of Sleep Medicine (WASM) and the World Sleep Federation (WSF), WSS states that its "fundamental mission is to advance sleep health worldwide." WSS aims to fulfill this mission "by promoting and encouraging education, research, and patient care throughout the world, particularly in geographic locations where the practice of sleep medicine is under developed. WSS represents over 600 individual members, 19 societies, and is located in over 50 countries. WSS organizes the World Sleep Congress every other year."

Phone: +1-507-316-0084

Email: info@worldsleepsociety.org

www.worldsleepsociety.org

Stay connected @_WorldSleep on Twitter and www.facebook.com/worldsleepsociety

Index

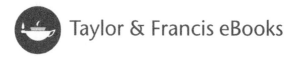

Taylor & Francis eBooks

Helping you to choose the right eBooks for your Library

Add Routledge titles to your library's digital collection today. Taylor and Francis ebooks contains over 50,000 titles in the Humanities, Social Sciences, Behavioural Sciences, Built Environment and Law.

Choose from a range of subject packages or create your own!

Benefits for you

>> Free MARC records
>> COUNTER-compliant usage statistics
>> Flexible purchase and pricing options
>> All titles DRM-free.

REQUEST YOUR **FREE** INSTITUTIONAL TRIAL TODAY

Free Trials Available
We offer free trials to qualifying academic, corporate and government customers.

Benefits for your user

>> Off-site, anytime access via Athens or referring URL
>> Print or copy pages or chapters
>> Full content search
>> Bookmark, highlight and annotate text
>> Access to thousands of pages of quality research at the click of a button.

eCollections – Choose from over 30 subject eCollections, including:

Archaeology	Language Learning
Architecture	Law
Asian Studies	Literature
Business & Management	Media & Communication
Classical Studies	Middle East Studies
Construction	Music
Creative & Media Arts	Philosophy
Criminology & Criminal Justice	Planning
Economics	Politics
Education	Psychology & Mental Health
Energy	Religion
Engineering	Security
English Language & Linguistics	Social Work
Environment & Sustainability	Sociology
Geography	Sport
Health Studies	Theatre & Performance
History	Tourism, Hospitality & Events

For more information, pricing enquiries or to order a free trial, please contact your local sales team:
www.tandfebooks.com/page/sales

 Routledge
Taylor & Francis Group

The home of
Routledge books

www.tandfebooks.com

For Product Safety Concerns and Information please contact our EU
representative GPSR@taylorandfrancis.com Taylor & Francis Verlag GmbH,
Kaufingerstraße 24, 80331 München, Germany

Printed and bound by CPI Group (UK) Ltd, Croydon, CR0 4YY

01/05/2025

01858521-0001